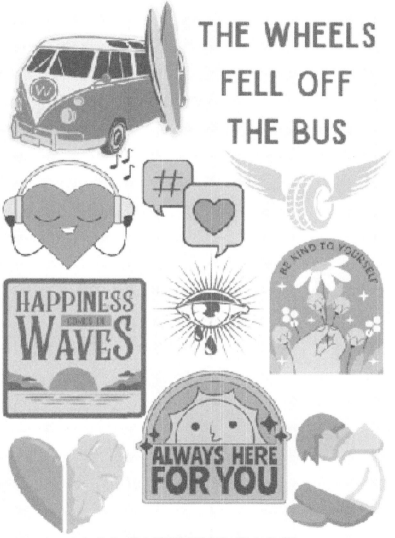

THE WHEELS
FELL OFF
THE BUS

MACKENZIE RICE

I owe this entire book to my beautiful wife, Rachel, that stood by me through the most trying times of our lives. The woman who saved me when I felt completely worthless. You were the light at the end of the tunnel for me and thankfully you weren't a train. I love you with every single piece of my heart, big and small. I am so thankful to be your wife, to be your person, to be your forever. Who needs luck when I have you as my partner in crime.

I also owe every single person that ever stood by my side on Tik Tok everything and more than I could ever say.

If it wasn't for my friends on the social media platform, I would not have found the medical care that I did and I wouldn't be where I am today. Each and every single one of you helped me through the darkest journey that I have ever dared to embark on and I love you all so very much.

Mackenzie Rice
Tulsa, Oklahoma
@Mer032511 & @Lesbianindieauthor
+Follow Me+
On Tik Tok

WHY THIS BOOK?

I won't sit here and tell you that this book will be a magical experience or that you will find any real value from it. I will, however, say that I hope my words can help someone, even if it's just one person.

I hope it can be similar to the light that was in my life during the horridly dark times that I was catapulted into. I hope it can encourage you to see your future in a positive way and give you hope for a better tomorrow, regardless of where you are right now.

I want everyone to know that proper and competent medical care should be expected and provided; for everyone, not just some. It shouldn't be just the simple fix situations that fit into the doctors standard box that get addressed and corrected. Some of us truly are zebras and not just horses. Doctors need to be prepared to handle us, just like they do 'typical' patients.

There were moments in my journey that I really wasn't sure if I would make it out. If I would reach the other side in one piece, or alive, for that matter.

I want you to know if you are going through a health crisis that there is someone in this world who cares and who has been on a similar path. That you aren't alone. That someone loves you and wants to do whatever they can to help. That there are options in this world besides giving up.

Health journeys, whether they are physical or mental, can be exhausting. Truly devastating for both the person experiencing them and the ones that love and care about them.

We all need someone that we can lean on when things are burning down around us. When the wheels have fallen off of the bus, sometimes even quite literally.

There will be stories in this book from my real life, traumas that I had to unpack and work through, even when I didn't want to. There will be unsolicited motivational quotes and life mottos that I used to get through the times when I didn't want to even get out of bed. There will be comical moments and sad stories, tears and even blood. (Oops, sorry. But that was a part of this horrid experience and can't be left out, as it is kind of what started it all. Trigger warning, there are photos at the end.)

Disclaimer

It will also be told in a partially fictional manner. The key elements are 100% as accurate as I can describe from both memory and copies of my medical records.

Certain names of individuals, doctors, and hospitals will be changed or left out all together. For legal reasons I can't expose certain names, even if I really wanted to. For that reason I have decided to write this a little differently than that of a typical standard memoir.

There is nothing worse than reading something that feels more dreadful than watching paint dry. I refuse to drag you through a boring memoir.

As you are reading this I want you to feel like you were there, standing with me. I want it to be easier to not only understand what I went through personally but to understand the absolute magnitude of what happens when we are ignored as patients. I want to highlight the tangible consequences of not listening to patients or completely disregarding them like they simply don't matter.

I want doctors, nurses and other medical staff possibly reading this, to see that, while they may be burnt out from things like Covid and dealing with insurance companies; we as humans and as patients are also dealing with the aftermath of those exact same things as well. While it may be in a different scope, the patient's viewpoint is just as important as the doctor's.

We as patients are met with the repercussions of your (doctors) actions that are beyond our control. We are bound to rely on medical professionals to help us.

Doctors are in the drivers seat that can either drag us from the nightmare that is chronic and even acute illnesses or hurl us into an emotional car wreck, while our illnesses are still there.

I truly believe deep in my heart 'most' healthcare workers do care and want the best for their patients. I do truly believe that there are a lot of amazing doctors in this world but that isn't what this book is about. This book is a reflection and exposure of the doctors who fail and further inflict pain upon patients with chronic conditions.

The ones who don't care, spoil the bunch. They are like cancer, infiltrating the system and spreading like wildfire. Their thoughts about people and their beliefs that we as patients are just making things up or pill seeking, will be the detriment to healthcare as a whole.

Through my medical journey, it became alarmingly clear to me, just how much cancer is in the medical world right now; just how horrible it has really become. Before my health crisis, I had no idea of the magnitude of the situation. It wasn't until I was standing in the pits of hell that I understood why so many people with chronic conditions feel the way they do.

I had always seen my mom go through emotional trauma with doctors. She has Rheumatoid Arthritis, Fibromyalgia, Ankling Spondylitis, Lupus and many more issues. It took her doctors years to believe her, ignoring her needs and tossing her here, there and everywhere. She has permanent, irreversible damage from being ignored.

I had seen family, friends and others that I cared about deal with these same ramifications but never expected to find that it was as bad as they said.

I hid in my bubble of, *"It isn't happening to me, so why does it matter?"* just like many others do.

Looking back, I really do wish that I had taken a stand for my mom. I was present at many of her appointments and never said a word. She needed someone to stand up for her, to back her, just like I did and you do as well.

We are all human beings with beating hearts. We all have a right to proper healthcare. We all have a right to be treated by a doctor who acknowledges our concerns.

We should all feel like we can be honest with our doctors and nurses, but we don't. We, the chronically ill, feel like we have to hide. Like we have to lie about what is going on with our bodies or leave out details because if not, we are making things up.

It's vitally important that doctors can see things from a different lens even if it doesn't fit into their go-to diagnosis. It is imperative that doctors don't force their patients into a box. That doctors don't jump straight to, "They must be crazy." or, "Here comes Dr. Google again."

We are all mothers, daughters, sons, fathers and so much more. We are people. We are human. None of us are just a number and we shouldn't be treated like we are. We should not be ushered in and out of a doctors offices, left more confused and more angry than we were before we walked in. We should not have to leave a medical professionals office in tears, feeling worthless and alone, but we do.

Language Warning

This book will have curse words as sometimes that's the best way to describe a situation. If you don't want to read something with F-Bombs, this isn't the memoir for you.

If you are ready and willing, let's go on this journey together, exploring the last 1,095 excruciating days of my life and a few moments of today shuffled in here and there.

Let's laugh, cry and maybe even get angry together. Grab a blanket, a cup of coffee, maybe some popcorn, put on Netflix for background noise or your favorite jams and let's do this thing!

CHAPTER 1

WHERE DO I EVEN BEGIN?

"Shit hits the fan so fertilizer can rain." -

Jackie Viramontez, Practitioner & Trainer

I have spent countless hours trying to figure out where to even start with my story. Analyzing everything that has happened over the course of the last 3 years over and over in my mind.

Trying to pick it apart in order to give you all some brilliant interpretation of the path that I have been on. To paint a beautiful and positive landscape, rather than focusing on all of the negative things that I went through. But the problem with that is you can't wrap dog shit up in a package, tie a bow on it and expect it to be a present. It just isn't possible.

My story was brutal. I will have scars and bruises for the rest of my life and I am not alone. There is an entire community of people in this world who share stories similar to mine. We as a society have to find a way to help others like ourselves. We have to find a way to make a change. We have to stand up and refuse to be silent.

My goal is take you on a walk with me through some of the most grueling and painful moments of my life. My goal is to show others like myself that there is a way to beat the system and we will eventually win, even if it takes forever. There is power in numbers.

And I want doctors and medical professionals to see that there is a second side to the story. There is a viewpoint that needs to be seen from the patients perspective.

You will see things in this memoir that I haven't shown to anyone. You will hear things that I haven't allowed myself to say out loud, even to this day.

I do want to put a trigger warning in for those who are not at a point in their journey where they can deal with feeling someone else's pain. My goal with this book is not to make anyone feel sorry for me or pity me. It isn't to make someone feel heartbreak.

But there will be parts of this path that aren't happy, that aren't beautiful and magical and kind. There will be situations where dark moments are addressed.

I would never want to create a harmful situation or make someone else have to relive their own medical trauma through mine. If you are not to a point where you can read about someone else's journey, that is 100% okay.

So... Where do I even begin?

To be honest, it's quite a trekking mission to go back to the start; to rewind my mind all the way to 3 years ago. While some of the details require a refresher, the beginning, I will never forget.

I was at work, standing with my boss, talking about a customer's car (I was a service advisor for a local car dealership) when I felt the horrid feeling that no woman ever wants to feel. I quickly realized that I needed to hurriedly finish my conversation and book it to my desk for some flow stogies. A trip to the ladies room was more than necessary at this point or I was going to start looking like the scene of a crime quick and in a hurry.

I really didn't think anything of it at the time, other than, great, here we go again. Another month of shedding my uterus lining and having horrible cramps for a week. Another week of feeling like I was going to eat the house down while curled up in the fetal position munching on my snacks. My own tears adding the salt to my sweet and salty personality.

In fact, I was actually kind of excited because I knew it was the one week of the month where I could eat whatever I wanted and not feel guilty.

I could blame my over indulging appetite for salt and sweets on the universe's natural course. And even had a semi built in excuse for my raging crankiness when I hadn't had quite enough coffee for the day.

Honestly though, I am never really cranky, ask my wife. I am more of the sunshine and rainbows shooting from my ass cheeks kind of person, but on the rare occasion that I didn't get enough sleep, I have my moments just like anyone else.

In fact, side story, one of mine and my wife's friends even gave me a cute care bear sticker that she got from Amazon that says, "Annoying Ray of Fucking Sunshine" for me to use for my water bottle or my laptop. I thought it was absolutely hilarious since I am both an exploding glitter ball of happiness usually and equally obsessed with stickers.

I'm not sure if it's the raging lesbian in me or the child that never grew up that resides deep in my soul, but either way, stickers make my heart happier than I could ever fully explain in words.

Taking a pause from my ADHD brain, let's get back to why you are actually here.

Several days went by, life seemingly normal at first. But as time went on things started to change. I began to realize that my monthly cycle wasn't slowing down; in fact, it was speeding up and at a rapid pace. I kept going on with life, working and being a wife and mom. Ignoring the warning signs and acting like they weren't happening.

I didn't have time to stop. I didn't have the money to stop either. I had to keep working, my family depended on it. Our bills weren't going to stop just because I had something going on with my body.

My wife had just graduated from nursing school and was still waiting on her new job to start, so money was a little more snug than I would have cared for. We were by no means destitute or living without any real needs, we just didn't have the money for some of the wants that would have made life feel a little less suffocating.

We also had just spent several weeks at the end of April going through a Covid nightmare where myself and my wife and all three of our kids were dying; or at least felt like it. I was lucky enough to have

"Covid Pay" at the time, however, it was not even close to what I was used to making and our budget and finances took a pretty severe hit.

I remember telling my wife, Rachel, that if the bleeding didn't slow down soon, I was going to need to find a way to go to the gynecologist.

In the back of my mind, I just kept telling myself that it would slow down and stop. I just kept lying and telling myself that I was just overanalyzing things and letting my stress get to me.

Several days very quickly turned into several weeks. I was standing at work one morning, typing on my computer. I felt myself start to get severely dizzy. It was an out of body experience that I really can't even begin to explain properly.

I felt like the world around me was spinning similar to how it is when you drink a little too much alcohol. The lights in the room felt like they were shaking and looked like shooting stars staggering all over the place.

I forced myself to take a moment to sit down even though my career world was burning down around me at the time.

If you don't know much about being a service advisor, it's quite the job. People are usually extremely angry when they come in. Their only form of transportation has now failed them and they are now late to work or don't have a way to get their kids to school.

Even if their car isn't falling apart they still aren't very happy because they are having to come in and spend their valuable time dealing with us. Not to mention, paying for maintenance and car repairs is much like ripping off a bandaid. While it is necessary, that doesn't mean it doesn't suck.

There were customers every direction I looked and a lack of staff that was only making the situation that much worse. People were running rampant around me, arguing and upset that they had to be there. The few of us working were dying trying to keep up with the demand.

It was also one of the hottest damn May days I had ever experienced since moving to

Oklahoma from Texas. Sweat was starting to accumulate in places that I didn't even know could sweat. My boob sweat even had boob sweat. It was brutal. In the automotive world we call that kind of heat, "swamp crotch weather". As disgusting as that might sound, it's pretty freaking accurate.

I knew that if I didn't take a moment to sit that I was going to come down on the raging hot concrete floors like a 50 lb. bag of potatoes. I hadn't been feeling overly great that morning, nor had I been feeling wonderful the last couple of weeks after Covid.

It felt like I just couldn't shake whatever had overtaken my body. Looking back and knowing what I know now with Covid and how it affects people, I realize that what I was experiencing was long Covid.

One of my coworkers stopped for a moment in the middle of the chaos and looked over at me. I can only assume that he was instantly worried when he saw that I had turned sheet white and had a bucket of sweat dripping down my face because he said, "Hey, Mack, you okay?"

I turned toward him, realizing that, no, in fact, I was not okay. I stood up, nodded at him, hoping he took that as a yes and then darted away from the service drive, up the stairs and to the bathroom. I really don't remember much of the walk to the bathroom, other than I know a few customers tried to get my attention, but I just couldn't formulate words to help them.

It felt like the entire room was spinning. It felt like I was going to pass out at any moment.

I remember stopping at the sink as soon as I busted the giant bathroom door open, the door slamming against the wall. I leaned over the counter, turned the faucet on, letting cold water fill into the palms of my hands.

I splashed my face, letting the water drip down my cheeks, my eyes darting to the mirror in front of me. *Woof. I look brutal.* I thought to myself, realizing that not only was my face sheet white but there were dark circles under my eyes and I looked similar to a Cullen from "Twilight", just minus the sexy and shiny part.

Internally I was hoping that the water would make the room stop twirling in circles even if for just a second, but it never did.

I stumbled over toward the bathroom stall and let my body slam against the toilet, exhaustion overcoming my entire being in a split second. I finally unzipped my pants and unbuttoned them so that I could use the restroom.

It was only then that I realized I had not only bled through my tampon but also through the pad that was lining my underwear. There was blood dripping down both sides of my legs and catastrophic things happening in the toilet that I won't even speak of.

All of this had happened in less than a couple of hours. I was in complete and utter shock.

I stood up, realizing that something was very wrong. I needed to go home. There was no way I could stay at work with my body internally attacking itself like this.

I cleaned myself up as best as I could and teeter tottered over to my bosses office, my head still spinning in circles.

Before I could even say anything at all, his eyes met mine and his face said everything I needed to know.

I could feel that he was seeing the exact same thing my coworker had seen just a few minutes before. The look of concern was painted all across his cheeks. I didn't even have to open my mouth before he told me I needed to go home.

I felt horrible. I knew they needed someone to be there helping with the service drive and I was leaving them alone to figure it out, but I didn't have a choice. If I stayed, I knew I was going to pass out, or worse.

I wobbled out to my car and drove myself home, which in hindsight, probably wasn't the smartest decision I have ever made but I couldn't think clearly.

Most of the drive home was a bit of a blur to be honest. I was just trying to get to my house so I could shower and change my clothes. I needed to come up with a plan of how I wanted to get help for this but before I did anything I needed to not feel like a walking oozing trash can.

I ended up calling my PCP and was referred to a gynecologist that was associated with my doctor's office. I really didn't want to make the phone call but I knew I had no choice. Obviously, acting like my problems were just going to dissolve into thin air wasn't working or making them go away.

I hadn't been to a lady doctor in years. In fact, the last time I had gone in for even just a check up was a couple of years after my daughter was born. My medical trauma starts well before just the last 3 years of my life. It began during my pregnancy and even after when I fell from a truck at work, rupturing my L5-S1 which eventually turned into Cauda-Equina.

During the labor and delivery of my daughter in 2010, the doctor delivering my daughter told me he didn't believe in episiotomies (cutting the perineum before birth to avoid ripping). I was young and had no idea how vital that could be or just how important that would eventually be for my pregnancy.

Unfortunately my delivery turned into a royal nightmare. My epidural was ineffective. Shortly after they placed it I realized I still had feeling in my legs and could move them as needed, but by the time the doctor listened to me, I was smack dab in the middle of delivering my daughter. There was no turning back now; no fixing the issue. I was already on the cusp of a dry birth. (A dry birth occurs when your water breaks and you still haven't delivered after 24 hours.)

Halfway through my labor, the doctor realized that the cord was wrapped around my daughters neck and she was starting to turn blue. He looked at me and while I was going in and out of consciousness, I will never forget him saying, "I need you to take a deep breath. The chord is wrapped around her throat. I have to get her out". I didn't know what he meant at first.

I took a deep breath as I was being instructed and before I knew it he was yanking on both sides of my lips, ripping me from front to back. I instantly felt like I was going to throw up, pass out and fall off of the table.

I wish it stopped there, but it only got worse. After my daughter was successfully delivered and I was still laying on the bed, trying to deliver the placenta, my doctor realized it just wasn't happening. He then proceeded to place his hands inside of me to grab the placenta and pull it out manually. (At the time, I had no idea that wasn't acceptable.)

In turn, two weeks later, I was hospitalized for endometritis. When I arrived at the ER I had a fever of over 104, my blood pressure was at stroke level and my hoo-ha was so swollen that the ER nurses had to use a pediatric catheter to even get a urine sample. I ended up having to have blood transfusions from the massive amounts of trauma and ripping. I was put on multiple IV antibiotics in the hospital for almost 2 weeks until they could get the infection cleared.

Flash forward to years later, my medical trauma only continued.

I was working for a dealership, once again understaffed on a Saturday in 2017. Everyone was running around like chickens with their heads cut off trying to make sure every customer was taken care of.

It was raining and hard. I walked onto our service drive which had bright shiny concrete floors. I pulled a truck forward to make room for other cars needing to be pulled into the garage. As I went to step from the truck I lost my footing on trash in a customers floorboard and slipped hitting my back against their foot railing. My feet hit the shiny concrete floors and slipped out from under me, with a vengeance I might add.

I slammed my ass directly onto the pavement and instantly felt one of the sharpest stabbing pains I had ever felt in my tailbone. I laid there for several minutes unable to stand up. I could barely move I was in so much pain.

It took a year for me to get help. I was forced into a workers' compensation claim that I would not wish on my worst enemy. I was tossed from one doctor to another until

I finally hired an attorney. It was only then that I was taken care of. They waited until I had lost all feeling to my legs. They waited until my entire saddle crotch region was completely numb and I was urinating and defecating on myself uncontrollably.

Doctor after doctor in the back pocket of workers' compensation almost let me live the rest of my life in a wheelchair.

I wasn't overly fond of going to the doctor after either of those experiences, PTSD playing a major role. It made every experience with doctors painful and scary, hence why I waited so long to get checked for my excessive menstrual bleeding in 2020.

****

The receptionist from the gynecologist office seemed surprised when I told her I had been on my period for just under a month at this point and felt it was necessary that I get in as soon as possible. They ended up scheduling an appointment immediately for the following day, which I quickly agreed to.

The next morning I walked into their office, instantly feeling out of place. I was standing in a room swarming with very pregnant women, which I was not. I checked in and then sat down, realizing that I stuck out like a sore thumb. Of course I had the female anatomy, the things necessary to need to be in this office, but I didn't look like anyone else. And it wasn't just that I wasn't pregnant.

Most of my life I have been different from other girls. I don't fit into the standard box of how a female should look and I never have. I have always chosen comfort over media's beauty standards. I have chosen myself and my sense of style over what I felt pressured into trying to be. I wear mens clothing because I am built like a brick shit house. I have wider shoulders than a line backer and have since I was little. I don't like makeup at all. It makes my face break out and it's tedious trying to keep up with, not to mention expensive.

I find peace in being me. Unfortunately, the world around me has never seen this as a positive thing and I could feel it with every stare venturing my way in the waiting room. I was anxious. I was on edge. It felt like the walls were closing in around me as the women around me continued to make me uncomfortable.

The nurse finally popped her head into the lobby and called my name, ushering me back to a room. We completed the normal nuance, "I'm gonna take your vitals, what medicines are you taking, when was your last pap smear, what brings you in today?"

I started explaining to the nurse what had been going on, telling her that I was bleeding like a stuck pig and nothing was changing that. She asked me how long this had been going on and when I told her just under a month, I thought she was going to fall out of her chair. She started frantically writing on her paper and then told me she would get the doctor and be right back. She pointed to a pile of gowns and told me to undress and get in one of them and the doctor would be in shortly.

After she walked out, I remember standing there holding up the atrocious gown, realizing that I had to remove my clothes and I would be essentially naked. Cool.

I took my clothes off and then like, every other woman, proceeded to try and hide my undergarments like the doctor wasn't about to have a speculum in my bits just a few moments later.

I sat down on the cold leather patient table, the crunchy paper stabbing my thighs and butt cheeks, pouring salt into an already open wound.

The doctor eventually popped her head into the room and asked if I was ready before coming in fully. She sat down and then we proceeded to discuss what was going on. She ended up ordering a series of blood work, a pap smear and prescribed me a high dose of Estrogen. I was to take 3 days worth of birth control on day one, 3 days on day two, 3 days on day 3 and then taper to 2 days worth for 2 days and so on.

I left the office feeling better, it felt like I at least had a plan. I was hopeful that the bleeding was going to stop and that life was going to go back to my normal. Boy, was I wrong.

CHAPTER 2

AND IT ONLY GOT WORSE...

"Get through today – you can fall apart tomorrow. Get through tomorrow, you can fall apart the day after . . ."

-Tabitha Suzuma

My life hasn't always been sunshine and rainbows. In fact, there is a lot of my life that has been excruciatingly painful. Moments where it felt like the sun had shriveled the fuck up, to be honest. Moments where I felt so entirely alone standing in a sea of people, feeling like I had no where to go or nowhere to turn.

Now mind you, when I say that, I am not trying to infer that I didn't have amazing and phenomenal people there for me. There are people who have done more for me than I could ever repay them for. I am incredibly indebted to some out of this world people.

But loneliness, trauma, pain… They don't have to just fit into a box. Just because we have amazing people there for us and just because we are thankful for the things we have been given and received, does not mean we cannot feel alone. It does not mean that we cannot feel like no one understands what we are feeling. It does not mean that we cannot feel like no one understands what we are going through.

We can still feel alone even when someone is standing right next to us. We as human beings can still feel unheard when someone is listening to our every single word.

There are things that I can't even share with you here that have changed the course of my life but the motto I have always told myself over and over is, "Baby steps. Little steps. One foot in front of the other. Just watch out for the IEDs."

It didn't and still doesn't matter what I have gone through or what I will go through in the future. I always tell myself, *"if I can just get to tomorrow, everything will be okay"*. And it almost always is.

That doesn't mean that the road to okay doesn't suck. Sometimes it fucking sucks. Sometimes there are tears and there is pain and it just sucks. There isn't a better word to describe it.

Sometimes tomorrow is actually next year and not today or tomorrow like we so desperately want it to be. But taking things in one small bite at a time sure as hell helps.

Approaching each catastrophic situation as one puzzle piece helped me digest all of the negative and process it so that I could move forward. Rather than focusing on the big picture, looking at all of the details, overwhelming myself; I have found it's easier to find one detail at a time. Focus on that, correct that and then move on to the next shit show that needs to be tackled.

Which is exactly what I did after I started taking the Estrogen that my doctor had prescribed me. It wasn't even 2 days after starting the high taper dose of medication that I started feeling like my insides were going to hurl up the back of my throat and out of my nose. I hadn't felt this nauseated since I had morning sickness while I was pregnant with my daughter. It was next level shit, to be honest.

I had tried to go back to work, to hoof it through the trenches of shit, but had quickly realized that if I couldn't keep my morning coffee down, then there was absolutely no reason to be there.

I finally gave up attempting to be at work and started harassing the doctor's office. I was messaging them and calling them relentlessly to let them know that the estrogen was making me feel like I had a demon trying to crawl from my stomach, but they couldn't care less.

By this point I would have paid someone to do an exorcism on me, just to see if it would make the waves of nausea slow down.

It was then that I quickly realized I didn't care for this doctor's office, as the response I received was, "go get some nausea medicine from Walmart and eventually it will go away." When I tell you the eye roll that occurred on my face as I was reading that message led to me penetrating the back of my brain, that is not an understatement.

I was shocked. The doctor's office had put me on a medication that was causing a severe side effect and the best advice they had for me was to go to Walmart and get some tummy meds. Cool story bro. It felt like a slap in the face, especially since I knew there were alternative options. They didn't care.

Several more days went by, the story getting that much more intense as the nausea had now turned into literal upchucking of my guts.

I called the doctor and messaged them again, explaining that the situation had gotten much worse and the over-the-counter meds simply weren't cutting it, to which I got back, "Your blood work is normal, your pap smear came back normal. Try Dramamine." As if I hadn't been taking Dramamine like a dope fiend since that was their only suggestion in their previous message.

They knew that and still ignored me. Still made me feel like I was a burden to them. That I was taking up their precious time for other people who had real problems.

I finally gave up, realizing that they weren't going to help me. I decided that the next day I was going to go to Urgent Care, it was my only option. I couldn't afford to keep missing work but I knew there was no way that I could work while I was still bleeding like a faucet and now I was projectile vomiting and dry heaving like a cat with a hairball every two-seconds.

That night, I went to sleep like my new normal, wrapping up two pads in my underwear and placing my nightly tampon. I took as much nausea medication as I possibly could and stopped to realize that I had now been bleeding for over a month.

My wife was starting to get angry at the absolute lack of urgency from my doctors. My family was starting to get upset. This was becoming ridiculous and at a rapid pace, too. It was June and I was still having issues; this shouldn't be happening, but it was.

I woke up during the middle of night, my body drenched in what I thought was sweat. I didn't feel hot, I felt cold even, my teeth starting to chatter. I got up and groggily walked into the bathroom, ignoring the giant mirror beside me and found my way to our toilet room, still half asleep.

I sat down and pulled my shorts toward my knees, realizing that it wasn't sweat I was feeling all over me, or sweat causing my shirt to cling to my stomach; it was in fact blood, lots and lots of blood.

I had it from my feet all the way up my back and down again. When I stood up and off of the toilet, I realized that there was a blood clot the size of my hand in the bottom of it. My underwear was bright red and also had a clot the size of a tennis ball.

I stopped, my heart was racing. I was in complete shock. I felt my stomach sink to my feet. I had never seen this much blood, much less, my own. I stood up, not even sure what to do, panicking. It was 3 in the morning. Everyone was asleep, where I should be.

I finally got my shit together and took all of my clothes off and showered. I realized that regardless of what was going to happen, I couldn't do anything in my current state.

I walked into the bedroom, realizing there was blood all over the bed, the sheets completely soaked through. It looked like a scene from "Unsolved Mysteries" in our bedroom. And that is not an exaggeration.

I didn't want to wake Rachel up, she had to work the next day and I knew she was exhausted. Our kids had to go to school and I had no idea who I could call at 3 A.M. to come get me and take me to the ER.

I finished cleaning up everything as best as I could and covered up my side of the bed so Rachel wouldn't roll on top of it. (I know that's disgusting but I really didn't know what to do at the time.)

I ended up putting myself to sleep on the couch, wrapping the pillows and cushions in giant towels, hoping that I didn't ruin everything we owned all in one night with my period palooza.

The next morning Rachel came out of our bedroom and found me on the couch, confused as to why I wasn't in bed. I explained what had happened and showed her the pictures I had taken. I showed her the mass casualty that had occurred on my side of the bed, her eyes looking as if they could pop from her head.

It was a real-life horror scene.

She was pissed at me, of course, wanting to know why I didn't wake her up, mad that I had gone all night without going to the ER and worried about what was going on with me. Why this was even happening?

It should not come as a surprise that I was in the car on the way to our local hospital shortly after that conversation. One would think that the hospital would be set up to help with my situation but that wasn't the case for me.

The ER, as all of you probably already know, through your own experiences, wasn't the most helpful. They did their series of tests and blood work, just as the gynecologist before had done and listened to me listing off the countless symptoms that kept adding to my growing list.

Once the tests came back normal, apart from my blood work, that was starting to show signs my red blood cells slipping, they ushered me out of the door with a referral to a different gynecologist.

The ER doctor stated that my red blood cell values were all lower than they should be but just a hair above needing a transfusion so there wasn't anything more he could do for me.

They didn't give me any real advice and essentially told me that if it happened again or if it got worse, to come back in. What was worse? They really couldn't be serious about that, right? Worse than hemorrhaging all over yourself and your bed?

I wasn't going to argue. I was exhausted. I had no energy and I was already starting to lose my mind dealing with doctors ignoring me and acting like I was making a big deal out of absolutely nothing.

It felt like all of the life was being drained out of me. It felt like I was being hung out to dry and told to just wait it out.

So I did just that.

I was already sick of seeing one doctor after another and really didn't know what exactly I was supposed to do since the ones I had seen so far, didn't seem to care.

I was essentially bleeding to death and even the ER didn't care. There wasn't anything they could do right that second. I wasn't having a heart attack or a stroke. I wasn't stabbed in my sleep or shot, so it wasn't something they could fix.

I remember thinking to myself, if the ER can't help me and my PCP and gynecologist can't help me, then who the fuck is supposed to be able to help me?

I called the next day and scheduled an appointment with the second gynecologist, telling them what had happened and referencing my latest ER visit. They scheduled me for my birthday, June 9th. I will never forget it.

June 9th rolls around and I still haven't stopped bleeding. Except now the relentless nausea and vomiting has turned into 20-25 lbs of weight loss in roughly a month and a half.

I walked into the doctors office, once again, feeling out of place. I tried to fix my eyes on anything and everything I could besides my nerves, my leg shaking and tapping, my foot pressing against the floor.

The nurse called me back and we exchanged similar conversations as I had with the previous office, rehashing and explaining everything over again now, for the fourth time. I felt like it was Groundhog Day. The words spewing from my mouth in a rhythmic and almost memorized state at this point. It felt like I was reading from a script, hoping to finally find someone who would listen.

The nurse was checking my blood pressure and I can't for the life of me remember what the reading was, but I do remember that it was high enough she had to call the doctor. She wanted to see if he still wanted me to stay at their office for my visit or if he wanted me to go immediately to the ER, again.

I was in mild pain but nothing bad enough in my opinion to warrant that high of a blood pressure. I essentially chalked it up to "White Coat Syndrome" and passed it off.

The doctor told the nurse, "No, I want to see her first." And then had the nurse take me back into a room to wait for him. He came in, a young guy, looking like he had just stepped out of medical school.

He was super charismatic, had great bedside manner, and told me that he wanted to do an endometrial lining biopsy since my ultrasound from the ER showed that my endometrial lining was thicker than normal. I agreed.

He and I discussed the medicine I was currently on, including the nausea and the weight loss that I had been having. His smile quickly changed from bright and big to non-existent. He explained to me that a thickened endometrial lining could indicate some pretty scary things and we needed to identify the problem as soon as possible.

He told me he would prescribe me Zofran for the nausea and was going to switch me to a Progesterone only tablet (with no Estrogen added) to see if that would help with the bleeding and the nausea. They did the endometrial lining biopsy that same day.

When I tell you that hurt, that is not a lie. Holy shit. That is one of the most uncomfortable procedures I have ever had where I wasn't asleep and had nothing for pain at all.

I won't get myself started on a rant, but it is absolute horseshit that a woman can have a piece of her endometrial lining chiseled out of her, like it's no big deal, with the expectation that pain medicine would not be needed. But healthcare for men is exponentially different. They get their balls snipped and next thing you know they have a month of pain medication. I just can't. I really can't understand that logic.

The worst part about the biopsy was that it got even worse as the day went on. The cramping turned into some of the worst contraction like spasms I had ever had. It was even worse than when I was in labor with my daughter, which is saying a lot.

Fast forward to a week later, I am still at home because I can't keep anything down. There is absolutely no way I can do my job. I can barely do what I need to do for myself and family. I have such little energy that it feels like I could pass out at any time and I am still bleeding.

By this point I had seen my PCP countless times, complaining of the weight loss, nausea and vomiting. Telling him about the blood loss, explaining to him that my fatigue was getting worse and worse as the days went on. He didn't seem that worried but referred me to a GI doctor anyway. He checked more basic blood work that had already been checked and sent me home.

It wasn't long after all of this that I received the phone call from my biopsy. It was normal. I was getting really sick of hearing "normal."

This time the doctor's office had changed their tune, telling me to keep taking the progesterone and eventually the bleeding would stop. By this time I was somewhere around 40-50 days of bleeding and no one trying to help stop it or do anything more than the bare minimum to find the cause.

I finally broke down, realizing that the bleeding was just getting worse and worse with no end in sight. I felt so lost, so abandoned. I knew I couldn't keep going on and on like this.

I scheduled an appointment with my PCP's second doctor, hoping that getting a new set of eyes on my issues would change something. I ended up having a mental breakdown to my PCP's office who finally listened to me. She sent me to another gynecologist within a totally different healthcare system and ordered additional lab work than what had already been preformed; all of which, normal.

While all of this was going on, I met with the GI doctor who set up a series of tests and different blood work than had already been done.

Everything kept coming back normal, normal, normal. But I was still losing more and more weight. They scheduled an EGD, colonoscopy and ultrasound of my gallbladder, all mostly normal apart from hemorrhoids and diverticulum.

I kept complaining, kept throwing a fit, kept telling them that this was not the quality of life I wanted or should be having.

I was up to 40 lbs. of weight loss by this point, food becoming something of the past. Every time I ate anything I felt like I would throw it back up almost immediately. My body even started rejecting fluids. I could take two sips and it felt like my stomach was going to explode.

I finally heard back from my GI doctor after harassing them relentlessly. I wasn't going to give up. I wasn't going to let this go. I needed someone to help me and I refused to keep being ignored.

They eventually suggested that I have something called a HIDA scan performed after frequent appointments.

A HIDA scan is a test that checks the functionality of your gallbladder to ensure it's working like it should rather than an ultrasound that checks for stones and sludge.

I had no idea at the time, but even if your gallbladder doesn't have stones or sludge, it can still have something wrong with it causing it to not work like it's supposed to.

The test is quite a doozy. You literally have to eat radioactive oatmeal or eggs and they watch the tracer dye that they put in your food cycle through your stomach, liver, gallbladder and intestines.

It is the wildest thing I have ever witnessed in my life. I told my kids when I got home that I was going to eventually become Spider-Woman when all was said and done.

As I was dealing with that, trying to get appointments scheduled, trying to get the nausea issue settled, I was still dealing with a bleeding issue as well that kept growing. It was all becoming steadily the most overwhelming time of my life.

I finally got in with the next gynecologist, who quickly did the same thing that everyone else had done. Test after test, lab result after lab result and everything kept coming back normal. I was starting to feel defeated, to feel like I was completely wackadoodle.

How could every single test come back normal and there be nothing wrong with me but I keep spewing from the top and bottom? Things weren't getting any better and I was starting to look like something out of "The Walking Dead."

My new gynecologist finally broke down and said, "I think its time to do a diagnostic laparoscopy. We need to get in there and see what's going on and why you still haven't stopped bleeding. I can't promise we will find anything but I can promise we will try."

I agreed, explaining to him that this felt like it was getting out of control. It felt like everyone was abandoning me. I was in tears.

I had now lost roughly 50 lbs. I was pale white, and my blood work was starting to come back worse and worse by this point. In fact, the new gynecologist called me after getting a few of my results back and said, "Mackenzie, I need you to go to the store and get iron as soon as you can. Your ferritin results came back and you are less than 2. In the 20 years I have been doing this, I have never seen a ferritin level as low as yours. Also, after reviewing your lab work, it appears you have PCOS but I still believe we need the diagnostic lap to look further into the bleeding issues."

If you don't know what ferritin is, it's essentially your iron storage. Iron is partially what allows you to feel energized. It is essential to how your body operates and when it gets as low as mine had, fatigue is extremely common, if not expected.

I felt a little relieved. It felt like finally something was starting to make sense and some of the puzzle pieces were starting to come together.

A couple of weeks later I had my diagnostic laparoscopy and when I woke up from my surgery the doctor told me I had endometriosis all over the inside of my abdomen.

It was on my bladder, my intestines, my ovaries, the abdominal lining, everything. He even had to take a small portion of my abdominal lining out because of how badly it had infiltrated.

The doctor told me he tried to get as much of it out as he could, explaining that some of it was not removable where it was located. I was in tears. I was so happy and so emotional. It was the first time my wife and I had been able to breathe. It was the first time for either of us to feel like we had found some sort of resolution.

We needed this win.

CHAPTER 3

FOOL'S PARADISE. PIPE DREAMS.

"Harsh reality is always better than false hope."

-Downton Abbey

If there is one thing in this life I have learned it is that we are all dealt a deck of cards. Everyone gets the same cards, shuffled different ways, paired for different hands. Some of us get luckier than others and some of us are forced to have one hell of a poker face.

Our lives may all be different but we have many similarities in a lot of ways to everyone around us. No matter who you are, what social status you are, or where you fall on the economic ladder, it doesn't change the fact that we are human beings on this earth that will experience trauma and pain in some way shape or form. No one is exempt from the shifts in life. No one is safe from the bad things that haunt or the misfortunes that can come.

We all have trials, traumas and tribulations that we must defeat. Obstacles are thrown our way, placed on our roads as bumps to trip us up. Some of us, unfortunately, are given more of a sinkhole than a bump, but I digress.

The biggest difference between our hand and the next is when the cards are dealt and how we handle what we have in our fingertips.

For a long time in this journey, I felt like I was dealt a shitty hand. I felt like I was given a different deck of cards than those around me. My path is and was much different from my wife's, my neighbor's or the strangers' down the road. But different doesn't and didn't mean better or worse.

It took me a really long time to come out of the darkness; to stop looking at things as if they were happening to me because I was a bad person.

For a while, it felt like this stuff kept happening to me because I had put some sort of bad karma into the atmosphere, that my good deeds had gone unseen.

I kept telling myself that there was something I had done, someone I had hurt, that I had to fix before life would stop handing me the shit end of the deal; over and over again.

It wasn't until recently that my mind changed, that I started to realize I had the wrong mindset. While I reserved the right to feel the pain, I needed to use it as fuel instead of letting it be my detriment.

I needed to use it to put a fire under my ass and stop laying on the couch, hoping for my life to change and wishing my lucky day would finally come; That I would hit the lottery without even buying a ticket.

It wasn't until recently that I realized everything I had gone through and experienced could be used to help others. I finally understood that I could use what I had seen as a misfortune for so long, as an opportunity to change someone else's future. I want everything bad that happened to me to be a learning lesson for others.

Looking back, there is a lot I would change about how I was seeing things. Hindsight is 20/20 they say, and they are right. Sometimes we have to view life from the rear view mirror to be able to see what we missed while we were busy in the driver's seat.

Several days after my surgery, I was still bleeding but like my doctor said, it was normal. I had been through a lot and my body was still purging all of the gross stuff that had happened while they were looking around inside of my abdomen and cleaning up the endometriosis.

I ignored the feelings I had in my gut that something still wasn't right and started focusing on the nausea and vomiting that still wasn't going away. I saw the GI doctor again and had my HIDA scan completed. It showed that in fact, my gallbladder was only operating at 17%. It was supposed to be no lower than 35% and anything under 35% meant I needed to have it removed.

My doctor called and said, "Good news, we found out why you have felt so bad over the last few months and why you have been losing weight. Great news in fact, we can fix this. We will get you scheduled for surgery. Someone will call you to follow up shortly. Also, your ferritin came back and it's still under 2, so we are going to go ahead and set you up with some iron infusions to get you kick started. The infusions should help with your fatigue."

I was mind blown. I was happy, don't get me wrong. It was such an incredible feeling knowing that they had figured out what was causing all of my weight loss, nausea and vomiting. But I still couldn't shake the fact that I didn't even get an apology, that there was no acknowledgement at all.

I had spent weeks going back and forth to appointment after appointment. The last visit I had with my GI doctor before my HIDA scan, I was told I should take anxiety meds. They put me on a low dose for abdominal pain and said that it would solve everything.

They blamed all of my issues on a nervous stomach. They almost had me believing that I was the problem. That I was getting too worked up about my health and life. I almost believed them and stopped trying. I almost gave up because they refused to hear me.

I left my appointment feeling like I was absolutely nuts. I couldn't believe that they were saying anxiety was the reason for my nausea and vomiting. I had worked a high stress job with 3 kids and a wife for years. Stress was my middle name and it had never made me feel this way.

I tried to explain that to them and they seemed like it didn't matter. It felt like it just went straight in one ear and out of the other. They had chalked me up to just another patient with mental health issues.

Had I stopped trying to get answers and had I allowed the doctors to convince me that my problems were just anxiety, I really don't know what would have happened.

I spent the next several weeks getting iron infusions done at the local hospital. Feeling absolutely horrible after each one, but knowing that I needed them to eventually get better.

A few weeks went by and I was scheduled for my gallbladder to be removed December 23rd, 2020. I will never forget that date because I kept joking with my wife that it was one hell of a Christmas present.

In my head I kept saying, "Oh well, at least after this surgery, I will finally be better and everything will be okay."

While I was waiting on my gallbladder surgery, the date slowly approaching, I started to realize that the bleeding wasn't going away. It had gotten better but was still there. I was spotting every single day, without fail and it had been more than enough time post surgery for it to stop. Thankfully, by this point, I wasn't hemorrhaging anymore or I would have probably died.

I called the gynecologist and told him and he recommended I take the Tranexamic Acid that I had been prescribed before and Ibuprofen. That was the only real suggestion he had. He told me that he wasn't going to do a hysterectomy, stating that I was too young and he didn't have enough to go off of, that he hadn't seen anything during my surgery to warrant taking out my reproductive organs.

He hung me out to dry, like all of the other doctors I had come across, again. I will give him a bit of credit that his attempts to correct the issue were more than the previous doctors I had been to. All of this was happening smack dab in the middle of Covid, which we all know, was a global crisis.

Medical care during this time was almost impossible to get. Doctors were shutting down appointments and refusing to see patients. Hospitals were overwhelmed by the amount of patients coming into the ER with Covid or Covid-Like symptoms. Everything was pure chaos.

I give him more credit than the others because while all of that was going on, he did try. He just didn't try hard enough.

What I felt he didn't stop to think about was that while he was dealing with his own personal hell, I was too. I was being ignored by him and so many others. I was being told that my health conditions had to wait because of Covid. I was being told that my issues weren't bad enough. It was all very overwhelming.

I was devastated. I felt like I had finally found someone who cared, someone that wanted to help me but now that he had found the endometriosis, he was abandoning ship. He didn't care that I was still bleeding and that a trip to the ER verified that I had blood in my urine. He just wanted me to go away. He didn't want to deal with me anymore.

I sat and wallowed.

I was so frustrated. Not only was he not helping me anymore, but it had been discovered during my diagnostic laparoscopy that my bladder was prolapsing and he didn't want to fix that either. He kept sending me to have pelvic floor therapy done, to which the Physical Therapist told me, "I really don't know why you are here. This is so bad I can't fix it with any training or exercises. This is a surgical matter. Your insides are literally coming out."

I was so angry. I was becoming infuriated at being unheard and feeling like no one cared. It felt like I was all alone and I had no medical team on my side that wanted to help me. I really wasn't even sure what to do. I knew I had to keep moving. I had to keep trying. But I was starting to lose hope, starting to lose motivation to keep going.

It felt like no matter what I did or where I went, that it was always the same end result. I was not only spending money at a rapid pace with all of my appointments, but the bills for everything I had been tested for and operated on were starting to roll in. My mailbox was starting to explode at the seams.

My disability at the time was intact but it was minuscule in comparison to what I had been making as a service advisor. If you didn't know this, most service advisors can make as much or more than you can make as someone with a college degree.

We didn't have the money for me to keep chasing my tail, to keep hoping that a doctor would stop and listen to me.

I finally broke down and scheduled an appointment with a urologist hoping he would take my prolapse issues seriously but he did not. He acted similarly to how my gynecologist was acting and ignored the fact that my bladder was trying to fall out.

My wife changed jobs during this time and was hired at a hospital as a surgical circulating RN. She eventually was promoted to the lead circulator for her department, which just so happened to be gynecology. Thank God.

One day, one of her favorite surgeons and her were having a conversation. She told the surgeon what I had been going through and the surgeon instantly said, "Have her call and get on my schedule. Let me see her, read over her records and I will do whatever I can to help."

Keep in mind that by this point I was still bleeding. I started bleeding at the beginning of April and it was now December. That's an incredibly long time to have a menstruation cycle without any real stopping in sight. Before this situation, I thought 7 days was bad. Seven days is a cake walk.

I turned around and immediately called her office, hoping that I would be able to get in sooner rather than later. Thankfully, her office had been told what was going on and she got me in right before my surgery for my gallbladder.

She reviewed all of my records and completed an ultrasound, verifying that I did in fact have PCOS but that was not necessarily what the issue was.

In fact, with all of the medications I had tried, she didn't believe it was related at all. She performed a physical examination and realized that yes, I was in fact, still bleeding.

She also saw my bladder prolapse and asked if I was okay with her trying a test to see what kind of prolapse I had and how bad it was. I agreed and prepared myself for feeling like a science project, yet again. (That doesn't fall on her.)

That is just how I felt after all of the countless visits to doctors and all of the poking and prodding that I had endured up to that point. She is and was an amazing doctor that I am beyond thankful for.

During her test she numbed my urethra and inserted a tube into it. She asked me to bare down like I was using the restroom and much to both of our surprise, I shot the straw/tube across the room.

It flew with such trajectory that both her and I jumped. I almost fell off of the table from being startled as badly as I was. It was quite comical to be honest. I couldn't stop laughing as she started scoffing and saying she couldn't believe that any doctor had ignored this and refused to help me. I think I even snorted.

After a few more visits with her and a few more tests, her and I came to the agreement that the best option was a partial hysterectomy. I had already had a child and was not planning to have anymore and I needed the bleeding to stop. I needed to go back to some sort of normal life.

While all of this was going on in the background I had also just had surgery to have my gallbladder removed, a total weight loss of almost 70 lbs. by the time they got my gallbladder out. They had let it drag on so long that I had gone from 235 lbs. to 165 lbs. I was starving. I hadn't been able to keep an entire meal down for months.

I was in the process of healing from surgery, trying to find things to do at home. I quickly realized just how bad I had felt before my surgery now that everything was starting to get better.

I finally was starting to feel more like a human and less like a corpse. It was the first time in months that I didn't feel like I wasn't dying inside and that I could do small tasks without being completely drained.

I rested up, trying to make sure that I could heal fast enough and well enough to have my hysterectomy. I didn't want to keep having surgeries. I didn't want to have to keep going through this same thing over and over. The song and dance was starting to get old.

It was becoming exhausting, starting to feel like my body wasn't even my own anymore but I knew I didn't have a choice. I needed my lady parts out so that I could finally be 100% again.

March finally rolled around and I had my partial hysterectomy. I was so relieved, realizing that this time, the bleeding really had stopped for good. It was an amazing feeling to know that I was finally okay. I was finally back to my 'normal' apart from standard healing after a surgery.

I had stopped losing weight and was finally starting to be able to eat again. The bleeding had finally stopped, completely this time. Healing from my hysterectomy was actually significantly easier than I thought it would be.

My surgeon told me that when she was inside of my abdomen, not only had more endometriosis grown back but my uterus, bladder and urethra were ALL prolapsing onto one another.

Had I stopped, had I listened to the doctors that I had talked to before, none of that would have been found; at least not in a timely manner. I would have continued going about my life, dealing with misery and embarrassing situations for absolutely nothing.

It finally started to sink in to me that I had done the right thing, that pushing onward was the right move. I knew my body. I knew when something wasn't right and even though I had multiple doctors tell me that there was nothing going on, or that my labs were normal or that the ER wasn't where I needed to be, I never gave up.

It gave me the confidence to know that I was the best and only person to be able to tell a doctor when something was wrong. It reminded me that this was my body and there wasn't a soul in this world who could tell me that I wasn't living through what I was.

Going through a medical crisis is crippling when you don't have a doctor on your side. It will debilitate you and make you feel like you are losing your mind. Even though you know something is wrong, if there is not someone who can help you, who will listen, it will tear you apart and fast.

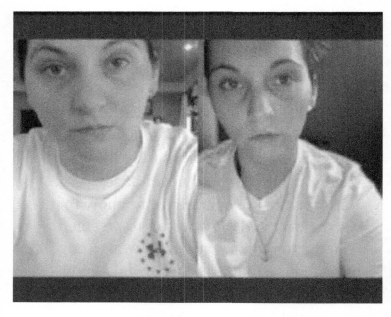

The image on the left was when this all first started back in April of 2020. The image on the Right is from October of 2020, roughly.

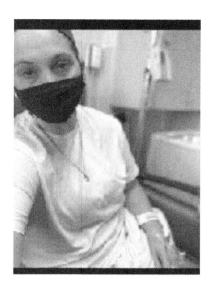

Photo was from approximately November 2020 receiving my first of many iron infusions.

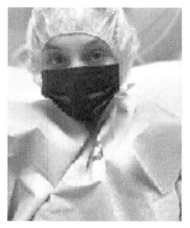

Photo is from before my hysterectomy March 10th, 2021.

CHAPTER 4

THE CALM BEFORE THE STORM

"The calm seas of Hell were only a break before the next storm."

- Jaxson Kidman

Have you ever had a moment in life where you felt like things were starting to finally come together? The world was starting to align for you. Everything seemed to be getting better and you were finally starting to feel peace, just to have it ripped out from underneath you?

That moment when life tears you apart, ripping you shred by shred, chewing you up and then discarding you like it's nothing is one of the most painful experiences life can hand you. It can happen in an instant. Life can turn on a dime as they say.

Life doesn't have to play fair. It doesn't have a rule book or a list of do's and don'ts it has to follow. It just does. And whether we are ready or not, it happens anyway.

I really thought life was starting to progress and move forward into a positive season. As I said before I had stopped bleeding, FINALLY.

The weight loss had stopped and I was able to eat again without feeling like it was going to come right back up. The sun felt like it was shining brighter and I was enjoying the fact that it was almost summer.

I felt rejuvenated. I felt like life had restored itself. My gallbladder surgery in December had finally healed completely and my partial hysterectomy from March was on the mend.

I talked to my disability and told them I only needed two more weeks and then I could go back to work, per my surgeons orders. I was so excited. Apart from a minor setback where my perineum decided to tear, everything was golden. For the first time in a long time it felt like I was approaching the finish line to being okay.

It felt like life was going to be magical again. I was going to be able to go back to my career. I was going to be able to finally try and work my way up the ladder and eventually be a Fixed Operations Director or a General Manager.

I was so excited thinking about how I would be able to work and my wife would be working also. We would finally have enough money to pay off the medical debt that we had been incurring but we could also go on a vacation; something we needed horribly. We needed a break from real life.

Life had been such a whirlwind of chaos, tossing us from one direction to another, without so much as an apology or even a warning. A vacation sounded absolutely mystical.

Until, once again, life decided to change our future. Life decided to stir the pot just a little bit more. It hadn't done enough damage.

One of my favorite sayings is, "I feel like I got run over by an 18-wheeler and it came back for seconds."

In fact, if you know me in real life, there is a very real chance you have heard me say something like that or a version of it. Dark humor is always how I have learned to cope with things that I don't know how to overcome.

I went to sleep one night in April of 2021 with what I thought was a tooth ache. I had been postponing having a tooth filled because of all of the issues that were going on with my health at the time.

It wasn't really an intentional postponement on my part. I just had so many other things going on that I couldn't take a second to address any of my other needs.

That night I experienced one of the worst pains I had ever felt in my life. I woke up between 2-3 A.M. crying; absolutely miserable.

I remember tossing and turning, trying as hard as I could to ignore the pain but it was getting worse. I took some Tylenol and Ibuprofen and then tried to lay back down but the pain was becoming unbearable.

It felt like someone had a knife slicing down into my jaw, stabbing me and then lighting it on fire. It felt like there was an electrical current running through my jaw, striking and burning me. The pulsations were so intense I wanted to die.

I really cannot explain to you just how horrible the pain was but I finally stood up, quickly realizing that I was not going to be able to sleep.

There was absolutely no way I was going to be able to close my eyes with this pain. I tried to be quiet but I woke up Rachel, who by this point had realized I was crying.

She asked me what was going on, worried and concerned that there was something more than just a tooth at this point. I went outside to pace, trying to take my mind off of the pain. I was hoping that if I paced, it would make it go away but it never did.

Sunrise finally came and the pain had finally slowed down some. I took more OTC medicine and then went to lay down, finally crashing and falling asleep for a few hours.

When I woke up, I realized that the left side of my face was not working, it looked paralyzed.

It looked like when I was diagnosed with Ramsay Hunt at the age of 21. It resembled that of Bells Palsy.

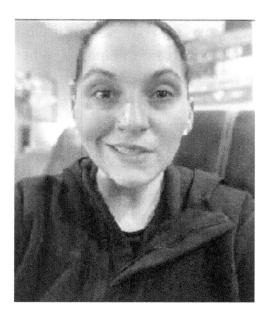

Picture was taken around April 2021. Left side of my face had an almost complete palsy.

When I realized what was happening, I instantly went looking for Rachel. I had to tell her what was going on. I was worried but honestly at first thought to myself, great, it's another Ramsay Hunt flair up. Just what I needed right now. Of course this would happen to me right before I am getting ready to go back to work.

Typical "Mackenzie's life" fashion to have something like this happen right when life feels like it's starting to change. When the light at the end of the tunnel is starting to become easier to see.

I kept carrying on for several days, hoping that it would just go away; hoping that if I let nature run its course that things would get better, but they didn't. Rachel was concerned that I had possibly had a stroke and kept urging me to seek care. I was hesitant after all of the medical trauma I had already experienced but knew I needed to do something.

I finally broke down and called my PCP. I told them what had happened and after a virtual appointment and a prescription for anti-viral medicines and high dose steroids, I thought I would be on the mend soon. That was the same treatment plan I had received years before when I was diagnosed with Ramsay Hunt.

I was wrong, again. It was starting to become a trend in my life, a repeating pattern of bullshit.

After another week or so, I called my doctor again. I let them know that nothing was getting better, at all. They turned around and scheduled a brain MRI, fear setting in for both them and myself that maybe I had a stroke the night I was experiencing severe left facial pain.

The MRI results showed that nothing was wrong, except something was very visibly wrong. My doctor ordered more steroids and then sent me along my way again. She told me that sometimes with Bells Palsy or Ramsay Hunt, they have to prescribe multiple high dose rounds of steroids to get it to go back to normal.

I took the next dose with hopes that it would just go away, but it never did. It just kept going downhill.

As time was passing by, the palsy was changing from a true palsy to more of a facial cramp. The cramps were becoming painful and my left eyelid was starting to twitch uncontrollably.

I contacted my PCP, for what felt like the thousandth time, and was told I needed to see a neurologist. This is where the journey really starts to become infuriating and this is where I really start to feel like my care took a nose dive off into an abyss of shit, to be honest.

That's saying a lot because up to this point, I had felt like doctors simply didn't give a shit about me. I had no idea it could get even worse, but I was about to find out.

I called the referred neurologist's office and was told that I could get an appointment but he had a 3 month waiting list. My PCP wanted a second opinion for MS since my MRI had come back all clear for no strokes but she had never seen facial cramps like this before.

During this time I was also referred to an Ear Nose and Throat doctor to check anything and everything else that could be checked.

The ENT, one of my favorite doctors, did everything she could. Her office not only got me in to see her in record time, she put a scope down my throat and then re-checked my MRI in her office just to make sure that nothing was missed. At least nothing that she could treat herself.

She couldn't find anything but quickly realized the TMJ that I had on the right side of my jaw was not really TMJ, it was more of a dislocated jaw.

I was sent to have more imaging done and then referred for physical therapy to see if they could help me get my jaw back into place. I wasn't able to go to PT though due to the fact that my face was semi frozen on one side.

During this time I started noticing that my ears were popping.

When the popping happened the best way I can explain it to you is that it sounded like a guitar amp being plugged in and then my ears being under water for several minutes, my hearing muted and muffled.

Other times, if I bent my neck a certain way or I moved just right, I would have really loud ringing in my ears, super high pitched like that of a dog whistle.

All of these super weird and random symptoms kept popping up more so than a bad batch of chicken pox.

They were here there and everywhere. I was starting to feel like Oprah Winfrey, "You get this symptom, and you get this symptom and this symptom."

All jokes aside, I really felt like things just kept getting worse. My disability company agreed to keep me on their payment list, realizing that with everything going on there was something deeper happening here.

None of this made sense though. None of the puzzle pieces were coming together for me. I felt so lost, so helpless and so alone. There had to be something that could make this all make sense; I just didn't know what it was at the time.

Around this time I finally broke down and started journaling my thoughts virtually on TikTok. At first, I really just created the TikTok as a personal journal. I wanted a place to talk about life, share my thoughts, share my journey, without being judged.

I needed a place to go that wasn't real life. Somewhere that I could share what was ping ponging around in my brain without having to share it with the people I knew around me. I felt like such a burden. I felt like all of these things kept happening and I was starting to look like a hypochondriac.

It felt like I was starting to look crazy or I was just making things up. I knew my wife didn't think that, I knew my friends didn't really think that, but all of this wild stuff just kept happening and I didn't know what to do or say about it anymore.

It was my life and I was living it but it felt like I was watching a TV show. It felt like my life was on season 9 and the writers were just making up the craziest shit that they could to get more viewers.

I felt like I belonged on an episode of "Jerry Springer" but for my health.

TikTok really did save my life. I will get to that more later but TikTok ended up being my saving grace. It was the place that

I found a community. It gave me a place to vent and scream and share the world inside of my mind without being judged, without feeling like someone was going to think negatively of me.

I kept waiting, posting here and there, bonding with others who were on a similar journey as mine. Meeting people who felt ignored, who felt like their concerns were not being addressed. Talking with them through the things that were happening to me and to them as well.

I started to realize just how many other people felt like they were being cast off onto some helpless island where doctors just didn't care anymore.

We were too much for them, too hard. We didn't fit into their box of normal problems and because of that, in these doctors eyes, we were all just crazy health hypochondriacs who needed to stop going to the doctor. We needed to get out of the way so patients with "real problems" could be seen and taken care of.

I finally was able to see the neurologist and my hopes were built up high that he would have an answer for me. I hoped that he would be able to help me with whatever was going on with my face. It felt like there was a constant mild charley horse in the left side of my face at all times.

I met with him and he said, "That isn't Bells Palsy or Ramsay Hunt. That's 'Hemifacial Spasms' and they are basically cramps that occur in one side of your face. They can come and go, they can get worse and they can get better. I have a fix for you. All you need is Botox and you are good to go. Hemifacial Spasms aren't curable but at least with the Botox, it won't bother you anymore. No one really knows why they happen; they just do."

Once again, I had a feeling of relief. I felt like I had found the thing that was going to make this all better and make it go away.

Wrong.

After dealing with my ridiculous insurance company who didn't want to pay for the Botox, I eventually was able to get the shots in my face.

Side note, that is one of the worst things to ever have to do. I don't really care for needles regardless, but having one come barreling at your face is not fun at all. 0/10, do not recommend. I honestly have to give women who get botox for cosmetic reasons major props. Their kahoonies are much larger than mine, that's for sure.

I tried the Botox several times. I kept giving myself false hope that it was going to get better. I kept feeling like maybe next time it will get better and it never did. The cramps started getting worse and the symptoms list started growing longer and longer.

It was around this time that I realized I could make my cramps stop by pressing on the back of my skull where it met my neck. I had been sitting outside in our patio chair when I leaned my head back against the metal bar of the chair. The pressure from the bar in the crease of the back of my head, relieved the cramp from my face. I was shocked. But when I sat up, the cramp returning.

When my wife got home, I told her what I had figured out and she was completely floored as well. She asked me if I could press on the back of my head and it would do the same thing or if it was just when I was in the chair.

I hadn't stopped to even think about that and ended up trying it. I realized almost instantly that it went away when I pressed on the back of my skull and pushed up. I ended up posting a TikTok of it and it went absolutely viral. I believe it has around 1.4 million views now.

My inbox and comments blew up almost instantaneously. I couldn't keep up with how many people were trying to help me.

I had every suggestion under the sun coming toward me about what it could be. But there was a resounding similarity of answers all pointing to "what if it's Chiari?"

At this point, I had never even heard of that. I had no idea what it was or that it even existed.

Finally, the neurologist I was seeing decided that he couldn't do anything else for me and he had no idea why the Botox wasn't working. He said he didn't think it was Chiari but he wasn't sure why I could make it stop by pressing manually on my skull. I showed him, hoping that by him seeing it in person, it would help. I really thought that him being able to see me make it stop, would be my saving grace. But it wasn't, at least not with his office. (Chiari is a malformation of the skull in the back of your head. It causes your cerebellum to sink or sag into your spinal canal. For more information, Google is a valuable tool. It's a lot to explain in such a short paragraph.)

He eventually decided that with the growing symptoms list that I was having and the fact that the Botox wasn't doing it's job, I needed someone different.

In fact, I will never forget when this doctor looked me right in the face and said, "I am not the doctor for you. This goes over my head and I have never seen something like this."

I was in complete shock. Utterly caught off guard. I was both worried and impressed.

I was worried because I had never had a doctor speak those words to me. Most doctor's approach things in a different way. Not all, but most…

I was impressed because it isn't often that you have a doctor say they aren't the right fit. It isn't often that a medical professional tells you that they are not qualified to help you. I was impressed because he didn't let his ego get in the way of my care and so for that I am thankful.

He referred me to a neurologist who sub-specialized in movement disorders in Oklahoma City. He informed me while I was in his office that because he was a sub-specialist, it was really hard to get into see him but he was a personal friend, so he would make a phone call for me.

Two weeks go by and I still haven't heard anything from my neurologist or the new office. I finally started to get a little concerned and placed a phone call to check the status. I was told that he had called them and that they have a really long wait list so it could be "a while" before I hear back.

I hung up the phone and called the movement disorder doctor, hoping to get a little more insight. I was told that their waitlist was eight months to over a year long. *A YEAR LONG…*

I didn't have a year to wait. I needed to get this fixed and needed someone to help me. I was fine with having to wait my turn, but a year? Things were getting worse and I needed to go back to work. I needed life to rewind or fast forward or just do something.

I was starting to have issues with nerve problems in my arms and legs, starting to experience incontinence and losing control of my ability to use my fingers like I had before.

I was starting to get extremely scared.

I have a family history of ALS, a disease that even before this health crisis, scared me.

While my neurologist said he didn't think this was ALS, he really wasn't sure. Those were his exact words.

I felt like if I had to wait a year and it was ALS, I was going to spend a year of unknowns with no help whatsoever, just getting worse and worse as time went on.

I continued posting on TikTok and trying to spend time with my wife and kids, hoping that I could distract myself from what life had become now.

I started really struggling with life, realizing that I was not where I wanted to be. I was having a hard time separating the good from the bad and starting to feel like the light at the end of the tunnel was a train and not in fact the sun.

I wasn't able to go back to work with everything going on. My laundry list of symptoms were getting worse and worse as the days went on. I was not only losing feeling in my arms and legs, I was having severe migraines, my heart rate was ping ponging up and down like a yo-yo flailing through the air.

Every time I bent down my heart rate would tank and I instantly felt as if I could pass out. There were so many symptoms piling on top of each other that I can't explain them all. My memoir would be the never ending story. (Instead, I have attached a list of my symptoms at the end for you to look over if you are interested.)

It started to feel like life was hopeless. I cried more times than I want to admit.

I would hide in the closet, dropping to the floor, sobbing and losing my mind. I didn't want anyone to see me losing my shit. I didn't want to admit that I was falling apart. I didn't want someone to see that I wasn't coping.

I sat in our bathroom toilet room (Yes our toilet has it's own room), screaming to myself, screaming at the universe, while no one was home. I just didn't understand why this was happening to me. I felt like I had to have been a horribly awful person in my past life or I was a bad person in this one and just didn't realize it.

I couldn't crawl my way out of my funk. The depression starting to settle deeper into my mind. I was depressed, lost and confused. I was tired of living like this, tired of feeling like this.

My health was making my depression that much worse, causing me to feel weak, making me feel like I was a loser. My health was making me depressed because I had no control over what was happening to my body and I felt like I had no one to help. I was drowning and every doctor around me was passing on an empty boat, just staring.

I needed something to change. I needed my mental health to change. I needed them to get my blood pressure and other symptoms under control that were beginning to spiral.

I needed them to fix my face so I could stop feeling like my face was going to twist off so people on the internet would stop saying I looked like "Popeye."

I needed them to fix me so I could talk about something other than my health. My entire identity had been stripped away and all that was left was everything that was falling apart. My breath had been yanked from my lungs, I felt like I had been sucker punched.

I was sick of having to take this medicine and that medicine, have this shot and that shot. I didn't want to be a science project anymore.

I finally decided to take matters into my own hands. I started researching what was going on with me, comparing MRIs of other conditions to that of mine. I started reading and teaching myself things as best as I could.

I continued talking to people, trying to understand and figure out what this could be. If doctors weren't going to help me, then I was going to figure out how to help myself. I didn't have a choice. I felt like it was either this gets better or I won't be here anymore.

As all of this was taking place and my symptoms kept getting weirder, my left collarbone started hurting, causing severe pain every time I moved it. It felt like someone had taken a brick and slammed it against my collarbone.

I noticed one night that my lymph nodes were also swollen and chalked it up to being related to my collarbone pain. I knew that when you hurt yourself or pulled a muscle, lymph nodes could react to whatever was going on around that area so I didn't think too much about it. I had so many other things to worry about that it just wasn't on the top of the list.

I mentioned it to my PCP, but just like everything else, I was told all was normal after having imaging done and ultrasounds of my lymph nodes. The doctors office said come back in six weeks and we will re-assess. But, when I went back and my lymph nodes had grown, I was told they were stuck in a reactive state and I didn't need to worry but that they would refer me to a breast doctor.

When I saw the breast doctor I was told I was just depressed and it was anxiety. I was berated by the doctor that I had seen and asked why I was even there. She annihilated me emotionally. She had me in tears. I was bawling. I left her office defeated and feeling like the world was cratering around me. Like I was being sucked into a black hole. Everything around me felt dark and cold. I was referred to her office by another doctor because their six week follow up appointment showed signs that things were getting worse and instead of talking to me about why they could be getting worse, the primary focus was that I was crazy.

It was one of the most disheartening moments of my entire life, if I am being completely honest. I have never felt so attacked.

The doctor that I had seen for my lymph nodes was a woman. While I know men can be sympathetic, I really thought she would be empathetic to my situation but instead, she looked at me like I was completely insane.

She proceeded to tell me that I needed to stay off of Google and I needed to essentially stop looking anything up. She told me that all I was doing was causing myself more grief and more anxiety and therefore making all of these weird things happen.

She didn't care that I have a strong family history of Non-Hodgkins Lymphoma. She didn't care that almost every single person in my family has had cancer in some way or another.

She couldn't even tell me why my lymph nodes were stuck in a reactive state. All she could focus on was everything outside of what I even came to see her for in the first place.

She told me that I needed to lose weight and then encouraged me to take depression medication. I was floored. I was completely taken aback, to be honest. I had never been treated like this in my entire life, by anyone, much less a doctor who was supposed to be there for me. A doctor that took an oath to help their patients, not harm them.

I drove home with my heart shattered and scattered across the floor of the doctors office. I eventually decided to take a break from trying to get help with my collarbone. Even though it was killing me and causing severe pain, my face and neurological issues were so much more important.

It was to the point that I was having severe heart rate fluctuations, almost passing out when I bent over, blood pressure readings at stroke level and so much more.

Finally after several months of posting about my condition and talking to countless people left and right about my brain MRIs a friend of mine on TikTok reached out to me.

They said they knew a neurosurgeon that might able to help me and wanted to know if I would be interested in talking to him and sending him my imaging.

I agreed and sent her everything I had, including the video of me pressing the back of my head to make the cramping stop. I would do just about anything to get help at this point and after all of my research, it looked like I had found a problem in the back of my skull where my cerebellum was located. I just knew that no matter what was going on, I needed someone to help me figure things out and clearly the doctors I had been seeing weren't doing that.

She messaged me back after getting all of the information that I had sent her and said that she herself thought something looked wrong. She had worked in healthcare for years and wanted to help in any way should could.

We talked back and forth for several hours before she told me that she would get back with me when she heard from her surgeon friend.

I was so thankful to have an outside look at everything that was going on. I would have waited just about any amount of time that it called for to have someone help that actually cared.

I was still waiting on an appointment with the sub-specialist that at this point felt like I would be able to see him when there was a cold day in Hell.

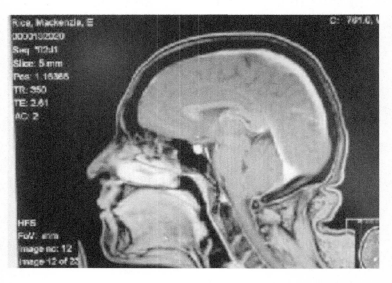

An MRI of my brain showing my cerebellum pressing against my brainstem. While it is not a typical true Chiari or Basilar Invagination (Google it.) There was not enough space for everything to operate as necessary. The decompression surgery opened up space. The fusion of my skull to my spine provided stability for my spinal instability caused my Ehlers Danlos.

CHAPTER 5

THE STORM.

"We must accept finite disappointment, but we must never lose infinite hope."

-Martin Luther King

Regardless of your religious beliefs, whether you have any or not, really doesn't matter for what I am about to say.

Faith. We must have faith. We must have hope that life can be better. We must not give up.

Life is too beautiful and too wonderful to watch it pass you by. There is beauty even in the painful moments.

I know that sounds cheesy. I know that sounds like some mantra that a self help guru shouts from their balcony with their beard hanging down to their chests and a joint laying on their lips.

But it so true. If we didn't feel the pain, if we didn't go through the storms, we wouldn't know what the sun feels like or that the warmth kissing our skin was a reprieve from the cold bitter air.

We wouldn't know what happiness is. We wouldn't appreciate the good times when life wasn't painful and wasn't dark and gloomy.

Realizing this was such an incredibly difficult task for me during all of my obstacles. Faith felt impossible.

I couldn't see past my own shit long enough to realize that in the grand picture of things "this too shall pass."

I was so focused on everything bad happening that I missed out on good moments. I squandered on times that I can't get back because all I could see was the cloud over my head. I felt like life just kept fucking me and I didn't want me to be happy.

I faked a lot of happiness. I put on my game face and I showed people what they wanted to see because I felt like I had to. I felt like when I showed my emotions and I showed people how I was feeling I was just being negative. I was letting everyone around me down.

I felt like I had to be this strong and fearless person or someone would think less of me.

I should have told someone. I should have tried harder to tell someone what was going on in my mind. I shouldn't have hidden that. I probably wouldn't have felt so alone in my head if I had. But I was so worried about what someone would say or think about me that I hid.

I even hid a lot of it from my wife. I told her a lot of what was going on in my mind but I hid a lot of the scarier parts. I didn't want to admit that I was at my rock bottom.

Also, side note; I can't delve into details but both my wife and I were dealing with other issues, important situations in our lives that had nothing to do with my health. Our worlds were blowing up around us and it felt like the air was being ripped from our chests.

I didn't want to burden my wife anymore than what we already had going on. I didn't want to be adding more and more stress to, what felt like, purgatory on earth.

I should have told her. I should have opened my mouth more. I shouldn't have let my pride get in the way of reaching out to her and others.

I want you to know that if you are the patient who is living a nightmare of their own, you must find a way to talk when things get bad. You must find a way to not shove yourself into a closet, hiding from the world.

It is 100% acceptable and necessary to feel what you feel. To express what is going on inside of your mind and what is happening with your mental health. Life is not always sunshine and rainbows. It is not dancing fairies and unicorns sprinkling glitter bombs everywhere. It is grueling and horrid sometimes. But we must keep faith. We must stop to smell the roses even when we are standing in pastures of cow shit.

If we are honest with ourselves and we share what's going on inside of our own minds, our view can change. We can start to see the bad things happening to us as just stepping stones to the next location. We can start to feel the wind blowing against our skin again and know that life will eventually be okay. Life will eventually change. Our course will take a turn and it won't always be this way. The wind will catch our sail and pull us back into shore.

As Martin Luther King says, "we must never lose infinite hope." If we lose faith and hope, we lose everything.

We can evolve and step outside of the bad things that happen to us. I truly believe that if we come together as a team and we lean on each other for support we can overcome anything in this life. We can knock any obstacle down.

That is exactly how I found my medical care. It was people who cared enough to help banding together that eventually fixed me. If I hadn't had those around me that cared enough to help I wouldn't be where I am right now.

The morning after I talked to my friend from TikTok I woke up to a text message from her telling me that her neurosurgeon friend, we will call him "Dr.

Wonderful" (because that's truly what he is) knew what was wrong with me.

I almost fell out of bed. I shrieked. I screamed. I scared the ever loving hell out of my wife. It was a chaotic moment.

I instantly messaged her back. I asked her what he thought it was. I asked her really every question under the sun to be honest. I was floored that he had responded so quickly and was so willing to help me.

After a series of messages back and forth she told me that she gave my phone number and information to the surgeon and he would relay the information to his team. He was out of state but not too terribly far from where I was.

I didn't even care. I would travel where ever I needed to go. The only reason I hadn't gone to the Mayo Clinic yet was for the simple fact that I would be going with no real plan. I would be seeing doctors who had never seen me thousands of miles away. I would be seeing doctors who would have to run test after test.

We didn't have the money or the ability to just up and drive or fly that far away. We had three kids to not only support but to make sure that we got them to and from school. We had to make sure they had what they needed and my wife had to work. We didn't have weeks to uproot our entire lives for me to have testing without a set in stone plan that I would get help.

It just wasn't feasible for us.

I was actually standing in Target grocery shopping for a couple of things we needed for the house when I got "the call". I will never forget because I saw the name pop up on my iPhone and I felt like I could puke. Why was the neurosurgeon calling me on the weekend? I knew it was him because of where the phone number was from.

I answered, pulling my cart off to the side of the aisle and said, "Hello?"

I heard his voice on the other line, explaining who he was; telling me what he had seen on my imaging, explaining how vitally important it was that I get in to see him or someone and fast.

He explained that my brain was starting to sink slightly and that the posterior fossa portion of my skull was too small causing compression on the area. (There is a lot more to that but I will spare you all the details.)

I stood there, my heart racing, his words circulating in my mind. I hadn't even really stopped to realize that I was standing in Target still. I was having this mind blowing conversation with a doctor I had never met and I wasn't sure what to think.

Everything he was saying was making sense but I still was just lost. How could this have been missed? If it was that serious and he was that concerned, how could this be happening?

He proceeded to explain to me that if I didn't have an Occipital Cervical Fusion with Posterior Fossa Decompression surgery soon there would be permanent damage. There would be irreversible consequences and the longer this continued on the worse those repercussions would be.

I felt my stomach sink to the floor as he started talking about me coming to his state and walking into the ER the following week to be seen. The reality of the situation was sitting on my shoulders like a giant dumbbell of weight.

The magnitude of knowing that every doctor I had seen for my symptoms ignored me and told me everything was okay; that I was just anxious, that I was just worried for absolutely nothing came crashing down on me like a ton of bricks.

The reality that some of the things I was experiencing may never go away because I was treated like a liar, like a hypochondriac, loomed over me like a giant dark cloud.

He wanted to get all of the imaging that he needed in one fail swoop. If we did it this way I could get the care I needed and the surgery he knew was mandatory without having to come back and forth out of state.

He said that I didn't have that time to wait. That I could get lucky and things could keep going the way they had or they could get substantially worse. My symptoms were getting worse already and my list was doubling, what seemed like every other day.

Nothing was getting better and I was starting to get very worried.

I left Target and I told my wife what had occurred. After talking about it we made the decision to trust this man. We decided to seek his care and made a plan to go to his hospital the next week.

I eventually heard from his office that they needed to schedule an appointment with me for insurance purposes to make sure they took my insurance before I drove all that way. I did everything that they asked. I followed all of their requests.

The woman on the phone I was speaking to started acting weird. She seemed frustrated. She seemed worried. But I brushed it off, thinking to myself, maybe you are just over analyzing things.

She proceeded to finish up my insurance information and then quickly got off of the phone with me.

I remember telling my wife, something felt weird with that phone call. Something about the conversation that I had with the woman just didn't feel *normal*.

I dismissed my concerns.

While I'm usually a pretty good read of character, sometimes I overthink and my anxiety creeps up. It makes me over analyze things that really don't need to be analyzed in depth.

I dropped it and moved on. I packed my bags and started a GoFundMe so that we could make the trip, pay the bills that I would have to pay for the surgery and make sure that everything was handled.

I was so ready to not be in pain anymore. I was so excited I started posting about it all over TikTok. I started a countdown to the day that I could get the surgery I needed. I boasted and was rejoicing that I had finally found the doctor to fix me. I was so relieved and overjoyed that I could finally share something positive with my friends and followers who had been navigating this horrendous journey with me.

My wife and I loaded up our bags into the back of our car and set on our way. We hit the highway and didn't look back. I was elated.

Until I got to "Dr. Wonderful's" office.

I checked in and the woman at the front desk looked nervous. She was callous and cold. She would barely talk to me. She acted like I had a plague.

I remember thinking to myself, *"This woman must reallyyyy hate her job."*

I filled out the paperwork she gave me and then brought it back. She didn't even stop to make eye contact with me; she practically ignored me while I was standing directly in front of her.

Before I had a chance to turn around and go back to my seat she informed me "Dr. Wonderful" was not there. He was on an emergency leave and I would be seeing one of their other surgeons.

I felt my heart sink. I had no idea what to think or what to do. We had just driven all this way to see a doctor who had a plan and knew what was going on. And now, I was being told the doctor wasn't even there. I couldn't understand why he wouldn't have called or texted me to let me know since we had been talking on the phone.

I sat down and told my wife what was going on and she supportively said, "Maybe this other guy will know what to do. A lot of times if doctors can't do what they need to because something personal happens then their colleagues will fill in for them. I am sure it will all be okay and everything will work out. I'm sure he must have had something pretty major happen for him to not let you know something."

Eventually the nurse popped her head out into the lobby and called my name. My wife and I stood up and walked toward her, following her to a room.

I sat down and proceeded to tell her everything. I told her about the conversation I had with "Dr. Wonderful" and told her about how I could make the cramping stop. I showed her as well. I went through every symptom and problem I had been having and explained how they were getting substantially worse as time went on.

She wrote everything down and then proceeded to tell me the doctor, we will call him "Dr. Dick", would be right in. I sat there with my wife, feeling extremely anxious and worried about if I was even going to like this other doctor.

I hadn't met "Dr. Wonderful" but I had talked to him on the phone. He had explained everything in depth to me. He was thorough and kind. I felt comfortable in knowing that he would operate on me. I felt like I had found the surgeon for me.

And now I was sitting here about to talk to a complete stranger about a massive brain and neck surgery. It felt so weird and scary. My nerves were on high alert and I felt like I could vomit. I remember sitting there, my legs tapping the floor violently, my mind racing in circles.

The doctor walked in shortly after the nurse left and dropped one of the worst bombs he could have ever dropped on me.

"Your MRI is normal and 'Dr. Wonderful' was wrong. There is nothing wrong with your scans and we are not prepared to help you. Where would you like me to refer you? It needs to be a hospital capable of this kind of surgery. Like 'Miracle Medical' or someone else besides us." (We will call them Miracle Medical to keep their name and privacy protected)

My heart tanked. My breathing stopped. Tears started streaming.

There was no way that what I was hearing was right. There was no way that I had driven all this way and told all of those people and done everything I had done to make this work, just for it to go this way.

I was flabbergasted. I was caught off guard. I was angry. I was infuriated. I was ready to punch "Dr. Dick" in the throat or the penis for that matter… But I didn't. Because violence against a medical professional is a felony and I am not cut out for prison life. Orange is in fact not the new black and it is not meant for my skin tone.

I had a "Legally Blonde" moment. I stood there thinking, "I'm sorry. I think I just hallucinated."

I paused and contained myself. I firmly disagreed with him and explained what "Dr. Wonderful" had told me and how he said the surgery would fix it. He stared at me blankly. He proceeded to inform me that he did not in fact believe the surgery would do anything and that even if it would help me, their hospital would not be the ones to do it.

I was thoroughly confused. His words weren't making sense. If he thought my scans were normal and everything was A-Fucking-Okay... Then why the hell was he wanting to refer me to a different facility for a possible surgery?

I lost my shit. I started ugly crying. It wasn't a pretty sight. I am talkin' full blown boogers, blubbering and choking, type crying.

My wife grabbed my hand and tried to console me and calm me down. I am so thankful she was there with me. If she hadn't been there to remind me to come back down to earth, I really don't know what would have happened. I could feel my heart pulsating in my throat and ears, my anger brewing and boiling. I wanted nothing more than to lose control, to absolutely spit in his face.

"Dr. Dick" proceeded to tell me that he would send a referral to 'Miracle Medical' but then said there was nothing else he could do for me and have a good day.

My wife and I were then ushered out of the room and filtered through the back door of the office so no one would see me crying. They didn't want to have to deal with me losing my shit in front of the other patients.

I don't remember much of the walk back to the car. I felt like I could upchuck my toenails. I had tears streaming down my face and the mask on my face felt like a coffin against my skin. I was hyperventilating and as close to a mental breakdown as I could possibly be.

I was one-second away from a "Lorena Bobbit" moment.

I sat in the car, quietly sobbing for I don't even know how long. My wife sat just as silent as I was.

Neither one of us knew what to do. She didn't know what to say to me; there were no right words. There was nothing that was going to change what had just happened in the doctors office.

It felt like we literally were living a nightmare, a never ending shit fest.

I knew that thousands of people on the internet were going to think I lied.

I knew that they were going to think I was a con artist and that I just asked for money for a fake surgery. I was so mad because apart from all of that I was still in the same boat. My face was still cramping and my body was still failing.

I was absolutely appalled.

I had no idea what I was going to do or how I was going to handle this. I had no idea what a referral to a different hospital was going to achieve or if they would even listen to me. I felt hopeless and lost.

The ride home was almost completely silent. I don't think I actually said more than 10 words in 5 hours. I stared out of the window my eyes focusing on anything and everything I could. I was sobbing and choking on my own tears and spit. I wanted to crawl into a hole and never come out.

I wanted to dig my grave right then and there. Place myself 6 feet below the ground and never come back.

My world felt like it had officially come down around me and I wasn't sure how to pick up any of the pieces at all. I felt shattered and scattered across the grass and left to rot.

CHAPTER 6

THE WRECKAGE. THE AFTERMATH.

"The world breaks everyone, and afterward, some are strong at the broken places." -Ernest Hemingway

Our darkest moments are when we really find out who we are as people. The darkness ironically shines a light on our character, integrity, and courage. It forces us to look deep inside of ourselves, to really find who we are. It forces us to push past every boundary we have ever thought would block us in. It thrusts us into territories that we never thought we would have to go.

When life is easy, most of the time, we don't have to try. Self reflection isn't mandatory. It falls by the wayside. When life is going according to plan we become complacent. We find our rhythm and out fear of rippling the waters, we get comfortable, we become stagnant.

It's only when life throws us upside down and back around that we have to, or feel obligated to, focus on changing ourselves to be the version we need to be. When life is falling apart, quite literally, we have no other choice but to sink or swim. Our brains are forced into fight or flight and we are bound to decide what we choose.

When the wheels have completely fallen off the bus and we haven't made it to our destination yet, we have no other choice but to find a new plan. When we have blown through plan A, plan B, plan C and are working on plan Z we find out who we really are as people.

The morning after my appointment out of state, I woke up, eyes swollen, looking like a dying raccoon. I felt hungover. I felt like I could turn right the fuck back around and put my depressed ass back into bed.

I didn't want to face the world. I didn't want to face TikTok or my friends or my family. I was so mortified and so disappointed.

I had honestly hoped that when I woke up the next day this would all just be one extremely realistic nightmare. I had prayed that I would get a phone call from "Dr. Dick's" office saying we made a mistake, come back. But that phone call never happened.

I paced the house for hours, crying and sobbing. I wasn't even sure what to say or how to say it. I needed to tell the people who had donated to my GoFundMe, Venmo, and CashApp that I wasn't in fact going to be having the surgery that I had told them I was.

I didn't know how to tell them that I was yet again starting this horrendous journey, all over again. I knew that someone was going to say I was a con-artist. I knew that someone was going to paint this picture of me being one big fat liar. I just knew it was coming and I couldn't blame them. I knew how it was going to look and sound.

I finally broke down and made a video. I tried to explain what had happened but also didn't know how to tell people "Dr. Dick" said "Dr. Wonderful" was wrong. I didn't really even know who to believe and at this point I was so confused and lost. Every doctor I had seen from my previous health systems up to this point had looked at my brain MRI and said everything was normal.

But "Dr. Wonderful" had looked and saw something different. Obviously something was wrong with me. I had all of these symptoms and health issues and problems. My face looked like someone had rung it out like a wet wash cloth. Clearly there was something going on and I truly felt in my heart like "Dr. Wonderful" had found my problem. Everything he said made sense.

Every journal article and document I had read about Chiari and similar conditions such as cranial cervical instability all pointed toward my issues. They all fit with what I had going on. I even discussed my imaging with another surgeon on TikTok who agreed I had a very small posterior fossa. How could so many doctors see so many different things from the same photo?

I posted the video, my stomach in knots.

I had a lot of really nice people respond who tried to encourage and support me. I had so many people reach out and try to be there for me. I also had a few people who verified my fears were accurate. A few of my followers/trolls accused me of being a liar and just using my community and friendship for money.

I couldn't blame them. I wasn't sharing a lot of the details and my video was extremely cryptic. I just didn't know what to say or how to say it. I felt like if I said the wrong thing, it would bite me in the ass. It felt like the world was watching my every move. I was just a puppet in my own life with no real control over what was happening to me.

That morning I called 'Miracle Medical' over and over again until I finally got ahold of someone. They had received my referral but hadn't gotten any of my other information yet. I was told to call back the next day.

I texted the friend who had helped me find "Dr. Wonderful". She was just as shocked as I was and offered to reach out to him for me. I didn't want to cross a line by talking to him myself.

A few hours later she responded saying that she had heard back. He said he was so sorry that he wasn't able to be there. He was flabbergasted that his coworker had done what he had done and said what he had said. She said he had to take an emergency leave of absence but that was all. I already knew that but something about this situation still didn't feel right.

I still felt lost and like I didn't have all of the answers. I had done my research on "Dr. Wonderful" before agreeing to come to his facility. I had verified his credentials and checked his medical license to make sure that he didn't have any horrible marks against him.

He was virtually squeaky clean and every single thing about him fit that he was a great surgeon. He had amazing reviews on every single website that I checked. Nothing about what he or my friend had said about him checked out as a lie.

"Dr. Wonderful" told my friend to make sure that I knew that no matter what I needed to go to 'Miracle Medical' and quickly. He let me know that my situation was dire and that it needed to be addressed as soon as possible. He was worried about me but couldn't help me at this time.

I posted another video shortly after trying to unpack more of what had happened with my situation without causing people to think I was even more of a liar.

All the while I was still trying to process what had happened to me. This was my life and I was living in it. While I felt like TikTok deserved an answer, I felt like I did too. My wife and family deserved answers.

Another one of my followers reached out to me and said, "I work for a company that helps people with crazy rare medical conditions. They find doctors across the US that are willing to help look over records and documentation. Their job is to help people find resources that they haven't been given before. I have a golden ticket. It means that I can give you this help for free. Would you like it?"

I am not gonna lie, at first, I was skeptical. I was completely worried that it was a scam. It sounded too good to be true.

At first I thought to myself, there is no way this is real and I am not responding to this person.

But as I sat and mulled over my current situation I realized just how lost I felt and how much I just wanted someone to help me. I finally broke down and responded to her message. The worst thing that was going to happen is that it wouldn't check out and they would, in fact, be a scammer.

It ended up being real. It ended up being one of the most amazing things that happened to me on this journey. It was a saving grace to some degree.

I signed up using the ticket I was given and gave them every medical document I had, including the documents from out of state.

The next morning I woke up to a call from 'Miracle Medical' stating that my referral was marked stat and that I needed a tertiary hospital. They got me scheduled and even scheduled me for approximately a week later, which in the surgery world, is almost unheard of.

It was slightly odd to me that a doctor who sat there and told me that I was perfectly fine would then turn around and mark a referral stat to a tertiary hospital.

If you don't know what that means, because at the time, I didn't either, A tertiary hospital is essentially a hospital on steroids. It is a higher acuity hospital that deals with everything under the sun; versus more of a hometown, basic hospital that deals with smaller more common issues.

As all of this was going on, I still couldn't shake that something felt off about what happened at the other doctors office. The puzzle pieces weren't fitting together at all. My spidey senses were on high alert.

Ironically within a day or two, I had an anonymous message from someone telling me what had happened with the previous "Dr. Wonderful".

The message explained to me that, "Dr. Wonderful" had shown his coworker "Dr. Dick" my videos from Tiktok. The videos showing how I could relieve the pressure on my skull, allowing my face to stop cramping and could even get it to work by lifting up the sides of my head as well. "Dr Wonderful" had shown "Dr. Dick" my imaging also and was looking to talk to them about my case. They agreed that they thought I needed the surgery but weren't 100% sure.

Come to find out, one of the people in the office had found my Tiktok and told someone higher up in the hospital what was going on. The hospital made the decision that because I had 28k followers roughly at that time, I was a giant risk for their name. The surgery was a much higher acuity than they felt comfortable having one of their surgeons perform, even if he was capable.

They made the decision to deny me care because they didn't want the bad press. They didn't want someone to be able to say that they did something they shouldn't have. They didn't want to deal with the aftermath if my surgery didn't go well. They forced "Dr. Wonderful" out of his job. The reason for his emergency leave is because he was fired.

The message I received explained that I still needed to get help. I still needed to keep chasing until I found a doctor that would help me.

I felt relieved but also infuriated. I was so mind blown. I couldn't believe that this was even real life. I couldn't believe that this was even really happening.

I had been through some fucked up events in my life and had overcome some of the most insane things you could ever even imagine but this by far was taking the cake as one of the most asinine moments I had ever lived through.

I was so taken aback. I didn't have the words to even express how I was feeling at the time. I could have put my hand through a wall.

A hospital that was supposed to be there for me and supposed to make sure that I was taken care of denied me treatment because of their name?

They denied me proper care because they wanted to save face? Are you fucking kidding me? A medical facility obliterated my emotional capacity over a stupid TikTok account. They ignored my physical well being over a PR issue.

I spent several days being unbelievably mad. I was not coping with my anger. I was sitting on it and brewing on it and letting it boil. I wanted to shove their words back down their throats and out of their asses.

I wanted to reach out to "Dr. Wonderful". I wanted to tell him that I was so sorry this had happened to him. I felt so unbelievably guilty. It was my fault. It was my fault that his entire world was being thrown upside down because he wanted to HELP ME.

This surgeon who had done nothing but try to do the right thing and be there for me, was now being punished because of me. He was now having to change his entire life because he tried to do the right thing.

I knew that nothing I could say would ever make it okay. I knew that I could never fix this and it felt devastating.

I couldn't tell the world what was going on, there were too many people that I cared about and respected that didn't need their names being drug through the mud. I was scared to talk about it because I had already made this huge disaster of shit all around me without even trying. If I told the world what had happened, I knew that I could be risking legal retaliation upon myself and my family, as well as "Dr. Wonderful."

I couldn't afford to have some big-wig hospital come after us because I opened my big fat mouth.

But I wanted to. I wanted to shout from the rooftops what had happened to me. I wanted the world to know that I wasn't a liar. I needed them to know that there was something wrong with me that still needed to be surgically addressed and now I had my proof. I had proof that the hospital out of state had screwed me over.

I wanted to tell the world what had happened so that this would never happen to anyone else again. I wanted to go after the hospital for damages, for refusing care to a patient that needed it. I wanted to sue their pants off. But how could I?

How could I leave more wreckage in other peoples lives to make myself feel better? I couldn't. I knew that if I approached a lawsuit, if I pursued medical malpractice, I would bring down the one person who had been there to help me in the process. "Dr. Wonderful" had already been forced out of a job and forced into uprooting their whole life.

A lawsuit would only make that much worse. And how was I going to prove anything with an anonymous message? Corruption runs deep.

So I didn't do anything.

I bit my tongue and I told my wife what was going on. I had to share it with someone. I needed someone to know what really happened. I needed to be able to talk through it and process it because if I had just held it in, I would have exploded.

The days went by and I finally had my appointment at "Miracle Medical".

I saw another amazing surgeon who looked at my stuff, looked at my videos and said, "Yes, you need the surgery. I don't do those kind of surgeries but they wanted you to be seen by someone ASAP. I will get you with someone who can help you."

I felt an instant relief. I felt a sense of calm. "Dr. Wonderful" was right. I wasn't wrong for trusting him.

I ended up finally seeing the sub-specialist who sent me on another tizzy though within the next few days. I had been waiting for several months when I received a call stating they had an opening and wanted to know if I could come in. Of course, I jumped on it, knowing that I hadn't met with 'Miracle Medical' at the time and that I had been waiting on this appointment for so long, I didn't want to just for go it.

I hadn't been reassured by Miracle Medical when I scheduled with the sub-specialist and just needed to get something from a doctor somehow.

The sub-specialist said, "I actually don't think surgery will fix you. I think what you are doing when you press on the back of your head is called a 'sensory trick'. You need anti-seizure medicine, it won't fix the issue, but it should help it." I was so damn confused. I was being tugged here and there and everywhere else.

It was nuts. Like complete and utter donkey shit, nuts. How could this many damn doctors see something so totally different, with a completely different course of treatment all at one time?

Who was I supposed to believe? Who was I supposed to listen to at this point? The information was more confusing than a damn corn maze to be honest. I would go one direction and the path would seemingly change before I could get to the end of the road.

Hearing the neurosurgeon from 'Miracle Medical' verify that he felt surgery would help, calmed some the noise, but not all. I still felt like there were too many different things being said by too many different doctors to really know what to do.

My saving grace was when I got a message from my golden ticket. They sent my information to a doctor in California who reviewed my records and my images. He agreed that surgery was necessary. He agreed that he saw Chiari, although slight, and that my posterior fossa didn't have enough space to allow my cerebellum to be where it needed to be and he saw a restriction of CSF fluid.

I needed that message. It sealed the deal for me that I was willing to take the risks of surgery. It made it clear to me that I needed to take this chance. Even if it meant that I could die, be paralyzed, or that it might not work.

If I didn't take the chance, I wouldn't know. I wouldn't know if I could be fixed and I would have been forced into having to take medicine over and over for the rest of my life.

I didn't want to be chained to medication. I didn't want to be locked into having to see doctors, specialists, and different providers day in and day out.

The neurosurgeon also mentioned something called Ehlers-Danlos to me prior to surgery (something that I had already heard about on TikTok from several of my followers).

He said with my laundry list of problems and previous health issues, as well as with all of my required surgeries, that it made it all fit. He wasn't a geneticist nor did he diagnose Ehlers-Danlos, but he was almost positive that I had it.

It would put every single puzzle piece together in one nice picture and explain all of the weird stuff that had been happening to me over the course of almost 2 years by this point.

He sent a referral to the geneticist but informed me that because there were only 2-3 of them in the entire state that it could take over a year to see one of them. This was becoming a pattern that I couldn't believe was real life. I couldn't believe that doctors we needed for our care were so hard to get into, so hard to come by.

It isn't something you really understand until you are standing there living it. If all you ever need in life is to see a primary care physician, the wait time is next to nothing. It isn't until things get wild, off the wall, crazy that you are faced with realizing, your options are limited.

We ended up scheduling an appointment for my surgery and I started preparing. I could feel the nerves in my stomach turning in knots.

The surgery that we discussed was an Occipital Cervical Fusion with a Posterior

Fossa Decompression. I shouldn't have looked up what the surgery entailed but curiosity killed the cat.

Just a heads up, if you are squeamish, I would avoid looking up that surgery at all costs. It isn't pretty. Especially if you are anticipating having it yourself.

While I was waiting for my surgery appointment to come I ended up finding a specialist close to my town who focused on Ehlers-Danlos.

I was astounded to know that he could get me in shortly after my surgery if I could pay out of pocket. He didn't take insurance so my appointment was going to be $250 to see him. It wasn't ideal to have to spend that money but it was a better option than having to worry about waiting over a year to see someone.

With my surgery coming up soon, I knew I didn't have the spare cash to get in with him. I had to focus my money on the surgery itself. I postponed making an appointment with him because I didn't feel like I really had a choice. But it was relieving to know that once we could make it work, I had found someone that could potentially help me. I was elated to know that I might finally be able to get the help I had been needing.

When you have a chronic condition or pain and symptoms that can't be seen, doctors typically won't take you seriously without a diagnosis on your chart.

Every time I went into the doctor and told them about new symptoms, I felt like I was being treated as a drug seeker; even though I never once asked for pain medication.

I felt like I was being treated like I was a Munchausen syndrome patient. Every single problem I had was almost always attributed to depression, anxiety or my weight. My BMI meant more to them than the fact that my face very visibly was twisted up like a pretzel.

I wanted to know if I had Ehlers-Danlos because if I did, at least then I could tell doctors why I had so many weird health issues. It would make the stars align so that they would know I wasn't just crazy.

I had done my own research. I knew that Ehlers-Danlos didn't have a cure, but I didn't care about that near as much as just being able to have something on paper that proved I was not psycho. That proved I was not lying or embellishing. That proved I was not a hypochondriac.

I had to make it all make sense. I needed medical professionals to start believing me and taking me seriously. It was my life that was hanging in the balance and they didn't seem to care. They had made up their mind about me and that was that.

CHAPTER 7

TWO SIDES TO A STORY.

"In seeking truth you have to get both sides to the story."

- Walter Cronkite

TRIGGER WARNING- MENTAL HEALTH DISCUSSION

Mental health is something that isn't talked about enough. It is so vitally important to be able to not only process and cope with life and its constant chaos but to be able to step outside of your thoughts and feelings and emotions. We have to learn to be able to look at a situation and realize that just because it's awful right now, doesn't mean than two weeks from now or a year from now, life won't change.

While I was on my health journey, navigating my own shark infested waters; I stopped being there for others in my real life. I reclused myself into a box and hid from what was going on around me. I was embarrassed and I felt like people were sick of hearing me talk about everything that had gone wrong in my life.

I was tired of being the person who had too much drama; that was too much. The problem is that most of the noise, was something I was just telling myself. Most of it was just the fear of rejection. I was so worried about people pleasing and having someone think negatively of me that I projected my own insecurities onto what others thought of me.

In doing that, I successfully pushed myself away from every single person I had ever really cared about. I did the normal texting, say hi to my friends. I didn't fully tear myself away from people but I wasn't allowing myself to tell them what I was really feeling.

I painted a picture that life was golden and even though all of this horrible stuff was going on, I was dealing with it and processing it. *"I was okay."* It was mostly all lies.

I even started to believe my own bullshit. I started to think to myself if I just fake it until I make it then it will be good. Which, I was right, it did all turn out okay.

But what I was wrong about, is that I should have been honest. I should have reached out to someone and told them I was not actually handling it. I got lucky. I got lucky that life never gave me my 13th reason why.

We as a community need to find a way to help those who need it. We need to find a way to help people who they themselves can't even admit they need the help. There are not enough resources in this world for people that need it.

When I was going through my health journey, I actually tried to get counseling and I was met with every road block you could imagine. From insurance not wanting to pay, to a list of doctors that had waitlists a mile long because they were one of the few who accepted insurance. To the inconsistency of available appointments and even to the crazy out of pocket costs associated with counseling if you didn't use your insurance.

It made me not want to talk to anyone. It made me not want to deal with the chaos and the cluster-fuck that was counseling. I was already struggling and having a hard time. I was already not coping and then adding road blocks just made that seem even more impossible.

This is a purely rhetorical question, but why is it that we as a society feel it's acceptable to make finding mental healthcare impossible to get? Why do we feel like people who are already having the hardest times of their lives and are in the darkest corners of life, should have to cross oceans and lands to get help?

There isn't an answer. It doesn't make sense. We are doing something wrong. The wheels have fallen off of the bus. We as a community have failed. And by we, I don't mean the people. I mean the systems set up and designed to make things as hard as possible for financial gain. The giant mega corporations that make sure you can't get what you need because it might cost them money; even though we are paying their outlandish monthly premiums.

That all mighty dollar is what we as a nation are worried about; capitalism before humans. It's actually quite disturbing.

And you don't have to have a specific political stance to feel that way. This isn't an issue of republicans versus liberals. This is an issue of Big Pharma and multimillion dollar corporations against regular every day human beings.

I only bring this up because I want to make it clear that I don't blame just the doctors for what happened to me. The entire system is set up to watch us fail.

The entire system is set up to put a barrier between the doctor and the patient, between the nursing staff and the human on the table.

Our doctors and nurses are burnt out from having to fight day in and day out to take care of their patients. They know what they can and cannot do to help the people in their offices and they are forced to put themselves into a box. They are forced to not look for zebras because the insurance companies think we are all horses.

It truly breaks my heart to see young doctors who waited and worked so hard to be healthcare staff because they wanted to help people, lose their fire and desire to be there for others through their own experiences.

It breaks my heart to see medical staff leaving their careers to find something else because it's better than dealing with the devil himself.

It is unbelievable to know that, "Suicide risk among doctors is said to be between 5 and 7 times that of the general population." according to the Indian Journal of Psychiatry.

It's my personal opinion, but I think suicide occurs because they feel an overwhelming amount of guilt that they aren't doing enough when there are times their hands are tied. (*This is for the good doctors.*)

There has to be a way to change this. There has to be a way to fix it. I don't have a suggestion because I am just little ole' me.

I am a girl from Texas who moved to Oklahoma and wrote a book once and used to be a service advisor/manager.

The people who are in the positions to fix this, to rectify what they have caused, can't see past the cheese. They chase it like the rats that they are not giving a shit what happens to anyone else around them.

Until something changes, life will continue on, just as it does every day. People will continue to keep seeking medical care that is limited to what the doctors and staff are capable of providing and their health will continue to suffer because of it.

Doctors, nurses and nurse practitioners will continue to leave the field out of pure exhaustion and fatigue. The burnout will leave an endless cycle of despair behind. We will consistently have to fight to get appointments with exorbitant waitlists because resources are limited. Young adults are already choosing other occupations than being a doctor and that will only get worse.

We will continue this giant rat race of shit over and over where we let the insurance companies dictate every single thing we do and decide our futures. Life will continue on and everyone will keep trucking along because they don't have any other choice.

Because... *they are like me.*

We are just the little people on the bottom of the ladder.

We might have a voice and we might have words that need to be heard but until someone at the top of the ladder decides to make a change, the cycle will continue. Until someone at the top of the ladder listens to the millions of us "little people", nothing will ever change. It's disheartening. It honestly shatters my soul. I would give my left tit to be able to make a change. I would give one of my kidney's and pinky toes if it meant that someone would listen to 'little ole' me'.

Mental health and physical health care should be a basic human right. It should be a given.

No one should ever have to choose between eating dinner every night or paying for their insurance. No human should ever have to choose between putting a roof over their heads or paying for their medications and care.

Yet, every single day, someone in America is forced to make those choices. To decide if they feed their kids or they get their medications. Clearly we are broken. Clearly the CEOs of these mega companies, need to start listening.

******

A few days before my surgery I got a phone call about my bill, the amount that would have to be paid in order for them to do the surgery. The surgery was not done in an "emergent" setting and therefore was considered elective in the insurance companies eyes.

My face being contorted, twisted and cramped up; my ever growing list of detrimental symptoms were being considered elective. I was mind blown. I couldn't believe that anyone could tell me that my surgery was a choice.

I guess with that logic, all surgeries are elective. (Insert Sarcastic voice here.)

I thought before all of this 'elective' meant cosmetic surgery; surgeries that you really didn't need, just wanted. I had no idea that surgeries a medical doctor said you needed done for health reasons could be considered elective.

Especially when the surgery they said you needed would fix mountains of problems you were having with your body; problems that could become life or death in an instant.

This is just one of the many, many examples that I could give you from just my journey alone and there are millions of others just like me.

There are people that as you are reading this right now are not able to get their procedures that they need, that would eliminate their pain. There are surgeries that would solve their problems but they can't have them because an insurance company says it's elective.

I just can't. I cannot fathom how that's even humane. I cannot fathom why insurance companies can tell me that I am allowed to have five counseling sessions but that's all I need. That's all they will pay for.

After those five counseling sessions if they haven't resolved my 30 years of trauma, unpacked it and fixed it, then I am on my own. *Wow.*

I cannot fathom that insurance companies can decide whether or not I need a medication. That they have the right to make any decisions about my care when they have never even seen me.

How can some doctor or nurse sitting in an office looking at paper work really make a decision about what is necessary or not?

Wow, is all I can say about that.

There are no words that explain the deep frustration I feel knowing that insurance companies have any right at all to control the outcome of our healthcare and it happens every single second of every single day.

CHAPTER 8

CLEARING AWAY THE WRECKAGE.

"Seems like the light at the end of the tunnel may be you."

- Steven Tyler

The day before my surgery I was a complete and total wreck. I was so nervous. I kept pacing in circles. I am quite honestly surprised I didn't put a hole in the floor with how much I kept walking back and forth.

I felt like I was making the right decision but everyone's back and forth, this and that, was clouding my mind and making me doubt myself. Making me doubt the doctors who had tried to help me, fearing that the doctors who said everything was fine, were in fact, right.

What if they were right and nothing was wrong and now I was having a surgery I didn't really need? All of these thoughts kept coming in and out of my mind, making me second guess everything; *confusing me even more...*

As we were on our way to the city, leaving my town behind, I couldn't stop shaking my leg. I was internally having a meltdown. It was almost sunset, the sun was shining across the horizon, little bits of purple and red intertwined with the yellow sun meeting the ground.

I remember thinking to myself that the sunset was beautiful, maybe it was a sign; a sign that everything was going to be okay. (I have always believed in signs from the universe as corny as that may sound.) I took a deep breath and reminded myself of all of the doctors who had agreed that this needed to be done. Finally calming down long enough to stop shaking my leg and tapping my foot on the car floorboard.

The morning of my surgery was even worse though. I didn't sleep hardly at all the night before. I was overwhelmed with nervous energy. I knew that no matter what this was the right decision but it didn't take away the fact that I felt like a gyrating worry wart.

We got ready and headed to the hospital. Check in went much smoother than I anticipated and before I knew it I was laying in a hospital bed, ready to go back for surgery.

It all felt very surreal.

Next thing that I knew, I woke up in PACU, the recovery department. I was in some of the most excruciating pain I had ever been in. The back of my head felt like someone had taken a hacksaw to it, my flesh burning and stinging every time I moved.

But I remember thinking to myself, what is that smell? One of the many symptoms that I had over the course of the year before was not being able to taste or smell.

I started instantly crying as soon as I realized that I could smell the oxygen from the cannula in my nose. I looked up at the lights in the ceiling and realized that I was not wincing, that my face wasn't cramped up at all anymore. My eye and mouth on the left side weren't working quite like they should but there was a very noticeable difference.

The tears streamed down my face something fierce. I was overjoyed. I was completely taken aback that things seemed to have been corrected. "Dr. Wonderful", the doctor from California and the doctors at 'Miracle Medical' were right. They fixed me.

The next few weeks were not very pretty. I was in severe pain. I couldn't find a comfortable way to sleep even with the wonderful body pillow one of my coolest followers sent me.

My neck was stiffer than a board and the neck brace I was in kept bothering me like no other. It was hot and made everything on me that much sweatier and uncomfortable. Keep in mind my surgery was in May so I was wearing this thing through the hottest part of the year. Not the wisest decision on my part or the best timing in the world. *(The surgery was the best decision I have ever made and I would do it a thousand times over again. However, wearing a neck brace when*

*it's hotter than a hoe in church outside would
not have been my first choice.*)

As the days went on, my face became
better and better; my other symptoms, most
of them at least going away completely or
becoming more manageable. Everything
was finally starting to feel like my old
'normal'.

The only real issue I was having now was
my collarbone. My left collarbone that had
been hurting and causing me pain, was now
shifted so far over it was sitting in the base
of my throat. It was protruding so much
that it was actually pushing my neck brace
to the side, making my head tilt to the right.
I even had a bruise on my jaw where the
neck brace had been rubbing too much.

I was determined that I wasn't going to
do anything about my collarbone though
until after I had healed from my surgery. I
was worried that I was trying to fix too
many problems at one time and my
neurosurgeon felt the same way. I put it on
the back burner and kept dealing with the
pain, realizing that eventually I could get
that issue handled too.

I ended up scheduling an appointment with the Ehlers-Danlos doctor shortly after the first month of my recovery. He was absolutely amazing. I have never met a doctor with beside manner like he has. He spent over 2 hours with me. I was shocked.

I was at the appointment with him for almost 3 hours in total. He tested me for Ehlers-Danlos and confirmed that I matched 9/9 on the Beighton Score. He also confirmed my suspicions that I had POTS and MCAS.

He explained to me that every single one of my symptoms were all intertwined and that they were all related. All of the surgeries, all of the problems, all fit together with Ehlers-Danlos and there were many other people out there like me that had similar but different journeys. I was completely mind blown.

He explained that Ehlers-Danlos could have played a significant role into every single thing I had been through over the last three years.

If you don't know what Ehlers-Danlos is, I would highly suggest reading about it on the internet. It is alarming and shocking at just how much it affects your body and how many problems it can cause with multiple systems within your body.

He explained that while some of these issues could have been unrelated to one another and separate issues, they almost entirely could be related back to Ehlers-Danlos as the culprit for why they had occurred.

Once again I felt a sense of relief. I felt like the world was coming together and things were finally starting to make sense. I finally for the first time, didn't feel like a science project.

I told my neurosurgeon about my appointment and brought him a copy of my report from the Ehlers-Danlos specialist. He wasn't surprised and was glad that I finally had the diagnosis I needed.

A few weeks later I followed up with a different PCP than my original for my collarbone because it was getting to where I couldn't swallow very well. I was tired of being ignored by my old PCP and knew something needed to change.

My collarbone was starting to feel like it was sitting in my esophagus, close to my vocal cords.

My PCP felt around, palpating the area and looked at it before saying, "I think you need an EGD but with you still healing from surgery, I highly doubt they are going to do anything about it right now. I will place a referral to an orthopedic surgeon but there is a very good chance they won't do much for you until you have been released from your neurosurgeon. I just want you to have a heads up."

And she was right. Unfortunately because of where I was in my healing journey, an EGD was completely out of the question. They did however do a CAT scan of my collarbone and verified that it was in fact dislocated superiorly. My doctor called my Ehlers-Danlos doctor and after consultation explained that they wanted to try something called prolotherapy shots before approaching surgery.

The surgery to repair my collarbone is a risky surgery and for someone with Ehlers-Danlos, it might not even be a permanent fix. To this day I have not done the prolotherapy shots yet.

Prolotherapy is not approved by insurance and they won't cover it, at all. Each shot is hundreds of dollars and I would need multiple shots for it to even work over the course of time.

There is also no guarantee that it will help me at all. The theory behind the shots is that it will strengthen and tighten the ligaments holding my collarbone and eventually shift it back to where it was supposed to be originally.

While I can understand the science behind it and I am willing to try it, I want to do more research and better understand what it's doing and how it can affect my body down the road.

Not to mention, I still am seeing 'Miracle Medical' for follow up post surgery care and would like to be released from them before I do anything else.

I am beyond thankful for my surgery. It gave me a quality of life back that I never thought was possible. My face isn't contorted anymore and I can taste and smell again. I am not having the same nerve issues I was having or the popping and ringing in my ears. My jaw doesn't dislocate anymore now when I open my mouth. I don't have a hunch back of Notre Dame on the base of my neck where my back meets anymore and so many other things have gotten better.

However, just like with everything in life, there is a consequence for every action. Since surgery I cannot turn my head right or left anymore and looking up is very difficult

I previously had to have a posterior lumbar inter-body fusion on my l5-s1 after I fell from a truck and herniated my disc causing Cauda-Equina.

My range of motion was already limited before my back surgery and now is limited even more from my neck surgery.

If you remember at the beginning of my journey, I worked for a car dealership. Cars were a huge part of my life and where I was headed moving forward.

Unfortunately, now I am unable to drive. Driving might be an option in the future, but as of now, it just isn't safe for me to be on the highway trying to change lanes.

Unfortunately, my disability insurance company decided that while I was unable to drive, I was completely capable of going back to work at a car dealership. Twenty other dealerships around my area beg to disagree. I have tried and tried and tried to find a job in my old profession, even looking into a parts counter job to attempt to return back to the working world; a world that I so desperately wanted to be in.

My Long-Term Disability company didn't care. They didn't see any need to continue my coverage. I was told by many, many different attorneys that, "Even if they re-establish your benefits, eventually they will cancel you again and this process will start all the way back over again."

I finally had been through enough. I wasn't sure what I was going to do, I wasn't sure how I was going to work with my modifications or what was going to happen with life but I finally decided if my life was going to change; I was the light at the end of my tunnel, not a train and not the sun.

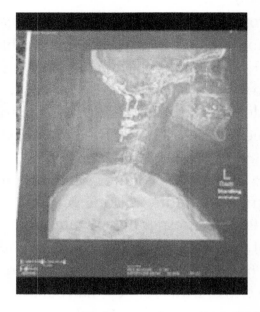

My X-Ray post-surgical procedure, June 2022.

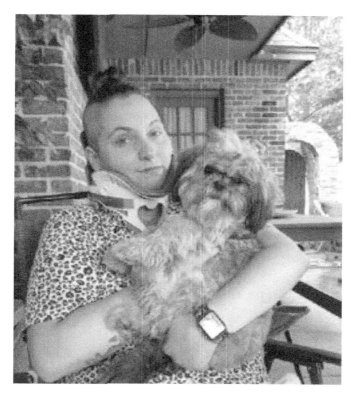

This was me the day after my surgery with my soul dog, Sophie. She was so excited to see me she couldn't hardly stand it. I almost started crying because I was so emotional at how happy she was.

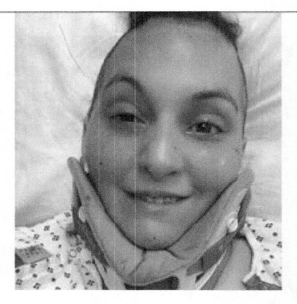

This is me the morning of my brain and neck surgery, May 25th, 2022.

CHAPTER 9

FINDING YOUR PEACE.

9 MONTHS POST DECOMPRESSION & NECK SURGERY

"Nobody can hurt me without my permission."

— *Mahatma Gandhi*

I wish I had the words; the right words. I wish I knew the exact game plan for how each and every one of you could navigate through your own individual storm. I wish that I had the secret to success when dealing with doctors, that there was a right and wrong way to handle each situation.

If I could write you a playbook for what to do, I would. But, I can't. I can't tell you what is right for your current situation or what doctor you need to see. I can't tell you exactly what you need to say to your doctor or to the medical professionals you are seeing, but I can do one thing.

I can tell you that standing up for yourself is vital to your success. I can tell you that no one knows your body better than you. You are quite literally the driver of your own bus. You know when the wheels are falling off and something needs to be addressed and no one can express that better than… *you guessed it, YOU.*

I can tell you that if you meet with a doctor and they don't seem to care; if they brush you off like a crumb on their shirt, they are not the right doctor for you. I can tell you that you deserve proper medical treatment and that while I do truly believe most doctors mean well, there are an overwhelming amount of doctors who don't. There are doctors in this world who leave us hanging to dry. We are literally at their mercy, unable to control our own health care and they ignore our concerns.

I can tell you that if you don't click with your doctor you absolutely reserve the right to fire them and move on. They are not your boss and you are not bound to utilize them. *(This is for the patients living in the US. I know other countries have different rules and guidelines for medical care.)*

Just as they can decide you aren't the patient for them, you can decide that they are not the medical provider for you.

Fuck loyalty if they cannot take the time to hear you. Fuck these doctors who think that doctor hopping is inappropriate. Excuse my French but if you aren't willing to really hear me, to listen to the silent screams that I am shouting, then you don't deserve my loyalty.

You can and must stand up for yourself. If a doctor is ignoring what you are saying and absolutely proving to you that they don't believe you, move on. While I know that it can be exhausting and it can be utterly overwhelming starting your process all the way over time and time again, it is imperative.

It is vital that you find the doctor for you. It is vital that you find the mental health care provider for you. They exist and they are in this world. Sometimes it can feel like trying to find a needle in a haystack but you need the needle. You need the doctor that is going to do what they have to do, what is in their power to take care of you or get you to the person who can help you.

You need a strong and compassionate PCP. Your PCP can make or break your health journey. They are your frontline warrior and while they may not diagnose everything, they are the doctor who will go to battle for you. If you don't have a strong PCP, I advise you to find one.

For a long time, I believed that my doctors were right. I believed that it was in my head or I was just making things worse than they really were. I believed that I needed to eat better, sleep better, and take depression medication.

While I can say that changing those things certainly helped, they were not my problem. Those issues were not what were causing my immediate chronic illness. They were not what were contorting my face, causing my lymph nodes to swell or what were making my collarbone be lodged into the back of my throat. They were not what was causing my heart rate to drop into the thirties, sending me into syncope. They were not what caused me to bleed like a water faucet or spew from both ends.

I might not be able to provide you a step by step "How To" but I can say that standing up for yourself is entirely possible.

It is imperative that we as a community stand up and tell the doctors who are not doing their job, that we will not accept their shit anymore.

Earlier I said, "Lil' Ole' Me" can't change things and I meant that. What I didn't say was that all of us, "Lil' Ole' Me's" can change things. If we stand up as a community and we take a stand, we can change the way the doctors, insurance companies and our country see things. There is power in numbers, there is strength in all of us that can change the way our world operates.

This is my call to action. My hope is we as a community, as a family that has been unheard for so long, can have the strength to take back the control. If we all stand up for ourselves and refuse to receive less than we deserve, the world can and will change.

It is single-handedly going to take all of us working together, banding together and working as a team to fix this mess that has been created.

"Lil' Ole Me" cannot change the world alone but As Martin Luther King Jr., said, "There is power in numbers and there is power in unity."

Doctors should care. Doctors should see us as the human beings we are. It is mind blowing that some of them become so desensitized to the world, so stuck in their own little box; that they forget we are the ones living through the nightmare.

If you have found a doctor that doesn't care, you are not a tree; you need to uproot yourself and move on. Do not let them get you down. Do not let them tell you that you are crazy and there is nothing wrong. Stand up for what you know is right in your heart. Stand up for the healthcare you deserve.

I believe in you. I believe in your strength and your ability to find the care you deserve. I believe you when you say, "Something is not right." And you need to believe you too.

The last bit of advise I can give you is have an advocate. It is imperative that you have someone who can not only go with you to your appointments but can have provide you someone to filter through doctors who choose to gaslight.

I would advise finding your own advocate. I know that sometimes that isn't possible; not everyone has family or friends who can or will go with them to every appointment. However, through my own experience it became very clear to me that the patient advocates in hospitals and insurance companies are not on your side.

While their job title indicates that they are there for you, in my experience, that is not the case. The patient advocates for the hospital are fire extinguishers and lawsuit prevention.

Advocates for insurance companies are money savers. Their job is to calm you down long enough and gaslight you into believing that they are there for you. In reality, their job is to figure out what the cheapest form of care is that can be provided and try to persuade you to do that instead.

Like I said though, this is just my personal experience. I am sure there are patient advocates out there that have been hired by insurance companies and hospitals that are genuinely good people.

But just like every other facet of life, you have to beware of the sheeps in wolves clothing.

*****

So who was I before all of this started?

I was a mother to three beautiful children embarking on their own journey's in this world. I have watched them grow and change, navigating the world and exploring. I am so proud of who they have become and where they are going in their lives.

I was a wife to one of the most inspirational people I know. I am amazed by her every single day.

My wife was previously married and endured a very painful and traumatizing divorce; a divorce that would have taken any normal human being down.

But it didn't take Rachel down. Instead it made her bloom, it gave her the water she needed to flourish. It was the fuel she needed to light her fire and set it ablaze.

She enrolled into a nursing program shortly after her divorce and graduated only a short 2 years later. She achieved the impossible.

I am so incredibly proud of her, of her drive to never give up. She has inspired me to keep going even when I didn't think it was possible or plausible.

I was a service advisor/service manager for a car dealership (Chrysler, Jeep, Dodge, Ram). I worked my ass off. I started out as a lot porter when I was attending college and was quickly promoted to a quick lane (oil change) service advisor.

A short year later I was then promoted to a retail service advisor and later promoted to a service manager position. I am a hard worker. I refuse to believe that I cannot do amazing things in this life.

I was a shot taker.

I have lived my life believing that we are the drivers of our own bus. We either ride off into the sunset, refusing to stop; refusing to veer off of our paths or we break down and stay there. We let the wheels fall off and plant ourselves into a rut.

I am the little engine that could and you can be too. Never let anything extinguish your fire. Whatever your passion is in life, whatever is on your bucket list, whatever goal or dream you have, DO IT. I cannot express this enough.

I never completed college. I let life get in the way. I let having kids and working a full time career take away from my drive but I refuse to do that now. I will go back to school and finish because I refuse to not finish something I started.

This journey has taught me that we have one life to live. I know that's a cheesy motto but it's very true. We are given one chance on this planet and we need to view that as an opportunity to go for what the fuck ever we want to.

You want to write that book? DO IT. You want to own that business? Work your ass off and DO IT. You do whatever sets your heart on fire.

Do whatever makes you the happiest person you know, even if everyone around you thinks you are crazy; even if everyone in the world says it isn't possible.

If you don't try, you don't know. And if you do try, it could be the best thing that ever happened to you.

Before college and living in Tulsa, I actually lived in Texas. My hometown is Lindale, Texas. I was born in West Texas and raised in East Texas.

My past is as checkered as a 50's diner floor, if I am being honest. I could write an entire other book describing my childhood and teenage years living in East Texas as a lesbian. *(I am sure you can imagine how that went.)*

So where am I now that my life went up in flames? Where am I now that the embers are smoldering and things have calmed down a little?

Well, I followed my own advice. I shot my shot. I refused to be taken down. I refused to let the doctors who steered me wrong, win. I refused to let the disability company that abandoned me, win.

I started applying for remote jobs left and right. I applied at every job under the sun. I was determined that I was not going to let life win. I was not going down without a fight.

Even if my life sucked right now, I was going to keep pushing and keep forcing myself into a better place. I was done hiding in the darkness. I was done feeling like life was out to get me. I was going to tackle life and knock it on it's fucking knees this time. *And I did.*

In between applying for jobs, doing things to help around the house and spending time with my wife and kids, I started writing. I typed my little heart away.

I let myself pour my soul into the words. I let the words drip from my heart into my fingers and through to my computer.

Pen to paper I finally started to let go of everything I had been holding onto, all of the dark energy I had been storing in my body.

It felt amazing. It felt like I was finally ridding myself of all of the negativity, the pain and suffering that I had been through over the last 3 years; maybe even longer than that.

I unpacked my trauma, one bag at a time. Day by day I started to feel more and more like a human being. I started to enjoy waking up again. The sun felt different. The trees and flowers looked even more beautiful. My world was being painted different colors, one-by-one.

It felt like I was watching a black and white photo merge into a color photo before my eyes.

Before I knew it I had written a book. I had finally finished a fictional suspense thriller and it was done. It had been a dream of mine ever since I was little. In fact, I started it in my journalism class when I was 15. My inspiration came from "Keeping You A Secret" by Julie Anne Peters.

When I was in high school I wanted to be able to read something that gave me the feeling of being included. I was a closeted lesbian for quite some time, navigating the world, lost. I felt so alone and just wanted to feel that I was represented somewhere. That there was someone in the world who was like me.

One day I was given a gift card to Barnes & Noble and my mom took me to look around. I found "Keeping You A Secret" and instantly chose it. It was about two girls coming into their feelings and addressing real life as lesbians. For once I felt heard, I felt like I could relate to someone or something around me.

I told myself that I would do that same thing for others like myself. I told myself that I would make a change in our world to hopefully give others like myself a place to call home, to feel loved and welcomed.

My goal with my writing after all of my life experiences is to not only write for the LGBTQIA+ community but to also write for every other minority there is. I want people that are disabled like myself to feel at home, I want people of different shades and colors to feel represented and welcome. I want to show the world that we are normal human beings and live very normal lives; that we are worth the time of day.

I always told myself that I would write a book, that I would chase my dreams and one of these days I would be able to call myself an author.

But as I got older, as my family got bigger and my work career got harder and more stressful, I put my writing on the back burner. I stopped putting pen to paper because I just didn't have the time or energy.

I gave up one of the things I love most in this world because of life. It was the easiest route for my bus at the time.

We all do it. We are all guilty of forgetting that we as humans need things that bring us joy. We get so fixated on chasing our careers and projecting ourselves into the next project that we forget we have needs too.

We forget that some of our needs aren't wants, they are actual needs; but we change them and make them 'wants'. We tell ourselves lies that we don't need hobbies, that we don't need to spend time with our friends and family. We tell ourselves that the most important thing in the world is our career, moving up the ladder and collecting more money.

I am beyond thankful that this journey brought me to where I am today. It was one of the hardest experiences I have ever been through and it was by no means easy. But it changed me. It gave me an opportunity to realize that I was the light at the end of the tunnel and not a train.

It gave me the opportunity to realize that I could change my path at any time. That I was not a tree and I was not stuck. I could do or be whatever I wanted to be.

It gave me a chance to realize that my wife and my kids came before anyone or anything else. It made me realize that I was focusing on the wrong things in life and putting entirely too much weight into being successful.

It gave me the chance to be able to say that even if just for one week, I was a best seller on Amazon's LGBT Top 100 list. That is an accomplishment that I never thought was achievable. I would have been happy with one person reading my book.

I may not be on the list anymore but I was and that is life changing for me.

It gave me the chance for my book to land in big name stores like Barnes & Noble and Books-A-Million. I overcame all of the odds against me and you can too. You are capable and wonderful and amazing. You have the power to take control of your life and make it your bitch.

It gave me the chance to get the remote job, a job that isn't near as stressful as my previous one. The job that I would have never gotten before this.

Sometimes in life, bad things happen to us but we have to perpetually tell ourselves over and over again that it isn't a bad life; it's just a bad day, or a bad week or a bad season. We have to find ways to reach out to those around us and seek help when we need it. We have to remember that even if the wheels fall off of the bus, there are always new wheels that can be put back on and staying on the side of the road, watching others drive past us, is not acceptable.

If you are experiencing something similar to what I was, I just want you to know that it's okay to not be okay. It's okay to feel what you feel and need a moment to get back up. It's okay to struggle; to dust your shoulders off.

But after you feel what you need to feel, you have to stand back up. You have to keep fighting and looking for the care you deserve. You cannot stand idle and watch your life burn down around you.

You are in the drivers seat of your own bus. If you have to plow through a few potholes or change a few tires, you can.

I have faith in you. I have faith that each and every one of you has a purpose in this world and path that will leave an imprint on someone else's heart. Never forget your own strength. Never forget that you made it to today and you will make it to tomorrow.

I also encourage you to find your voice. Speak your concerns to your doctor. If they ignore you and you are forced to move on, to find another; **go back to your original doctor**. Once you have your diagnosis and you find the doctor meant for you, **make your old doctor listen.**

Go back to the one who dismissed you and stand up for yourself. Take back the power. Explain to them in a mature and civilized way that they failed you. Make the doctor who brushed off your concerns hear you. It may not change them, it may not matter, but if we all start taking a stand and expressing when they were wrong; I can promise over time it will start changing the world.

If only one person stands up, doctors inability to care, their lack of compassion and blatant disregard for us, means nothing. If one person says something, that person is just crazy and proving that they were anxious or depressed.

But if we all take a stand, if we all start using our voice to make a change; then eventually these doctors will see that they are in fact the problem. As I said before, there is power in numbers. There is power in taking a stand for yourself and refusing to be a walking mat. I encourage you to face those situations with grace and poise.

I am by no means encouraging violence or blatant disrespect to any doctor or medical professional.

However, there is absolutely no reason we cannot speak with precision and tell them just how wrong they were. There is absolutely nothing wrong with looking them in the eyes and making them acknowledge that they fell upon the easy route. They didn't do their jobs and they need to hear that. They need to know that their abandonment affected us greatly.

The last bit of advice I can share that I learned through my journey in this nightmare is that you must network. You must reach out to those around you who have also experienced these things, who might have the ability to help you. If I had never reached out and asked for help, had I not shouted at the roof tops that I needed help; I would not be where I am today.

People can be kind. There are people in this world who want nothing more than to keep you from experiencing the pain they have had to endure. There are people in this world that will go to the depths of Hell to help you. There are people who would do anything to keep you from having to walk into the darkness alone.

Do not ever let yourself feel like you are a burden. DO NOT let yourself forget that there is still kindness and love in this world, that there are people who love you and care about you.

Never forget that sometimes asking for help, reaching out to a community like you, is the only way to survive. And if no one has told you today, I want you to know you are loved. You are cared for more than you could ever know.

I love you all, with all of my heart. We are in this together and even if the wheels have fallen off of the bus, myself and so many others will be there to help you change the tire.

SYMPTOMS LIST I CREATED FOR DOCTORS THAT WAS IGNORED:

*****None of this will be grammatically correct as it came directly from my notes pad on my iPhone and is exactly what I provided to EVERY ONE of my doctors:*

Symptoms:

Hemifacial spasms
Periodic sharp stabbing jaw pain that's excruciating
Arm pain is worse when swallowing, coughing, or with movement (putting hair up in a bun-movement makes it burn)
Armpits feel like I have done pushups, when I have not.
Facial weakness/spasms. I can use it but not the same as I used to. Different than true palsy.
Arms fall asleep while asleep almost every night.
Legs fall asleep. Saddle crotch goes numb.
Severe debilitating fatigue that's progressing.

Water type noise in left ear
Ringing and popping in ears when I bend my neck (both sides) (sounds like when you plug in a guitar to an amp. Super loud pop and then ringing that follows)
When I bend my neck sometimes my eyelid twitches (left side)
I can press on the back of my skull to make my face relax, doesn't fix it but helps relieve... as soon as I let go it cramps back up.
As time has gone on, when I press on the back of my skull or lift up on it to make the cramp stop, it now makes me dizzy, nauseous and out of it temporarily.
Loss of equal sensation in left side of lips, nostril compared to right
Difficulty swallowing at times feels like the left side of my throat stops working/something blocks it.
Also causing breathing issues in my sleep. Have woken up several times choking for air. Happens awake too when I cough sometimes.
Double vision/blurry vision in left eye at times.
Tongue seems to stop working at times, makes it hard to speak and words get slurred
Pins and needle feeling in finger tips, as well as loss of feeling and control in hands and arms at times.
Muscle weakness at times. Feels like I got a tetanus shot and can't lift my arms (both hands and arms (Both hands/arms)

Arms will burn with use (feels like workout when doing simple tasks like stiring or putting hair up)
Sometimes it feels like it's cold outside and when you come in, your hands and fingers don't want to work)
Random tremors in hands and arms.
Restless legs almost always (feels like static on a tv almost) constant need to move my legs.
Insomnia/Can't sleep.
Severe Charlie horse cramps in legs.
Weird tingling, pins and needles feeling, itching in my nose randomly. Full nose, not one sided.
Itching on chest, in under arms. Red spots that look like petechia show up where the itching is sometimes (feels like hard marbles under the skin)
Loss of taste or smell unless it's very strong/potent (salty, super sweet, spicy)
My voice changes, I've also lost my voice for a solid day.
Incontinence in my sleep both bowel and bladder (is happening frequently now)
Bowel incontinence while awake int mint (getting worse, happens almost daily now)
Horrible headaches that pound and pulsate, starts at back of head with pressure and gets to where I can feel it in my ears. Feels like blood or water pulsating in my ears. Feels like electric shock down my spine sometimes. Starts at top of spine and shoots down to the base of my spine. They have gotten much

more consistent and worse since botox. Only thing that helps is laying flat on my back. Moving in anyway or any activity makes it way worse.

Symptoms seem to be worse when standing or keeping my head up, if laying down, symptoms are better. Except the restless legs which are worse.

Cause severe insomnia without Gabapentin and Artane.

Water retention even with water pill and BP meds (drinking water daily too and magnesium pill)

5-10 lbs weight fluctuation over time.

Constipation without Linzess. (No solid bowel movements hardly ever. Mostly liquid.)

Urinary hesitancy (sometimes it takes 10-15 seconds to be able to pee even though I feel the urge.)

Different vitals in each arm. (Left and right read way different, even when taking them back to back.)

Right arm turning red/blue/gray/cold int mint. Feels like I have a tourniquet on.. pressure and fullness.

Burning, shooting, deep pain in right arm.

Swollen lymph nodes in right armpit. Verified on ultrasound, grew over a time frame of 4 months.

Inconsistent blood pressure readings with 2 BP meds and water pill. (Some high and some normal low)

Tachycardia

Low heart rate drops(happens frequently), nausea, dizziness, lightheaded, fatigue, cold body temp and sweats. (Temp drops to 96 and then goes back up after symptoms resolve)
Heart rate changes 30-50 bpm just from standing and walking a couple of feet.
Severe whole body-aches and flu like symptoms (armpits and chest muscles hurt bad)
Bending over causes heart rate to drop significantly and then shoots back up upon standing.
Arms fall asleep while I'm sleeping, both sides. Happens almost every single night, position doesn't matter
Red spots like petechia showing up everywhere
Blood pressure keeps going up and up no matter how much medicine I'm on.
Hands turn yellow off and on now, won't wash off with soap, rubbing alcohol, or acetone
Easy bruising; bruises showing up everywhere and no injury occurring
Severe joint pain all over body
Entire right side of body is swollen and has edema. I have photos to show it.
Ended up in the ER believing I had a heart attack; have labs to show; bloodwork had changed but was told not to worry and sent home with BP still at 140/107.
Severe exhaustion that's getting worse.
Lumps under collarbone (think they are lymph nodes) itch horribly off and on. Red spots

show up there but not sure if it's from itching breaking blood vessels or the spots just appearing on their own.

Family history of lymphoma, heart issues, cancers, autoimmune issues.

ER visit for chest pain and high BP. Bloodwork changed also. I have

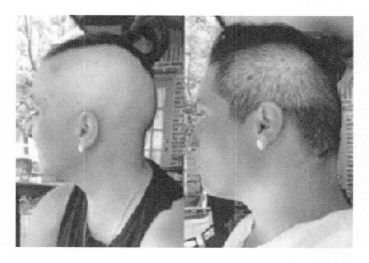

Comparison of my head before and after surgery. The swelling has gone down significantly since the photo on the right was taken.

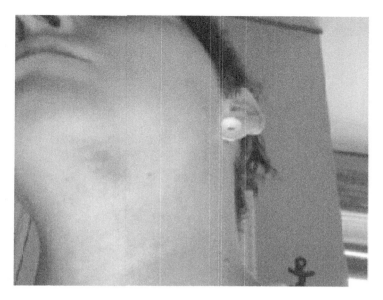

The bruise under my jaw from my neck brace rubbing due to my superiorly sublexed collarbone.

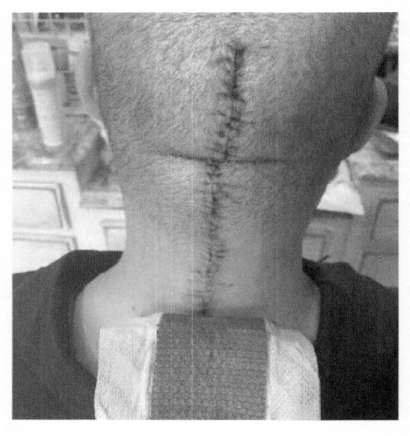

This was my incision a week or so after surgery. The bandage had come loose and I was able to see it for the first time.

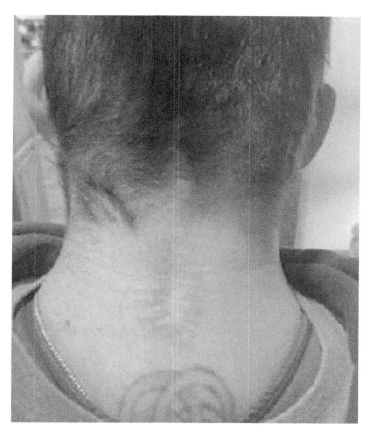

My scar fully healed January 2023. Scarring like this occurs commonly in Ehlers-Danlos.

A LETTER TO THE DOCTORS WHO DIDN'T TREAT ME:

"I have learned now that while those who speak about one's miseries usually hurt, those who keep silence hurt more." — C. S. Lewis

For a long time I couldn't find the right words. I felt lost in how to handle approaching each one of you.

I felt like my words might roll in one ear and out of the other, leaving me feeling even more frustrated. I knew that if you didn't agree with my feelings then I could potentially walk out of your office feeling even worse than I did when I first entered.

My fear ripped me apart. It fueled my inability to write this memoir. It created doubt that I could even come up with the correct words.

But, that changed.

I refuse to hold onto the anger. I refuse to be the one who has to carry the weight on my shoulders anymore. I refuse to be seen as a liar with anxiety. While I may have anxiety, that is not the causation for my issues and I refuse to be told that it is.

I approached one of you face to face, wanting to talk about my health and all of the signs that were missed and you dismissed me. You tried to act like you did nothing wrong, like a coward. You had and still have the power to help others. You could have helped me and you didn't.

I hope that you can understand, I only wanted closure and peace for my own heart while you were worried about legal issues. You only heard "lawsuit" and shut down. I never spoke those words and I don't plan to pursue it either.

I wanted to feel validated and acknowledged that mistakes had been made. I wanted an apology that I never heard and will never hear. But that is okay.

I hope that moving forward you can find it in your heart to help the people who see you after me. I hope that you never let someone suffer the way that I did. I hope that you never again force a patient to run out of your *office crying because you refused to hear them and kept demanding it was just depression. I hope that you can find it in your heart to reevaluate your decisions.*

The first time I walked out of your office crying, before our appointment was even concluded, I felt like a failure. I felt crazy and accused of having only mental health issues. I couldn't stand to be in the same room with you any longer. I knew that if I stood there and let you continue to berate me, to degrade me, I was going to lose it. I was not going to give you that control and I was not going to continue an appointment with someone who didn't want to actually help me.

Leaving your office this time, felt euphoric.

I walked out feeling proud, with my head held high. I haven't stopped smiling ever since. I regained my power and strength, I took my life back.

I refuse to ever settle for doctors like you ever again. I refuse to be told that I am just anxious or depressed when something in fact is wrong. I refuse to let a doctor be the driver of my health. If you can't respect me enough to hear the words I am saying, to genuinely listen to me and communicate with me, you are not the right doctor for me.

I will not harbor anger toward any of you anymore. What I will say is that I hope you read this and know that you failed. I hope that you can see, not everyone fits into your tiny box of diagnoses that you try to put them in. I hope you know that there are people you have utterly given up on that needed your help. I hope you know that there are patients who have refused to see another doctor, even when they needed it, because they were ignored, just like me.

I hope you know that you could have destroyed my life. You could have driven my bus straight into a head on collision, if I had let you.

I hope the "Dr. Dick" reads this and feels 2 inches tall. I hope that he realizes the magnitude of his decision to refuse to treat me and to block a doctor from helping me. I will forever live with permanent nerve damage because of the time it took for someone to help me. I will never be able to fully smile correctly. I will always have incontinence at times and I will continually *have to deal with the ramifications of your ignorance.*

You changed my life and not for the better. You took an oath to do no harm and you did. I have found my strength. I have found my voice and I will not stand for being subjected to poor medical care. I will not allow myself to be treated the way I was for the last 3 years, ever again.

I speak not only for myself but for every single patient who has been ignored by a poor doctor. I speak for every human being who hasn't found their strength yet. I speak for those who are scared to use their voice. I speak for every patient who feels that proper medical care was not given to them. I speak for every single patient who had to suffer for YEARS before a good doctor came to their rescue.

I hope that you yourself do not ever have to experience what we as the patients have.

Have the day you deserve…

TO THE DOCTORS WHO WERE THERE FOR ME:

"Dr. Wonderful", I owe you my life. You gave me the second chance I so desperately needed. You are the reason I am here today and finally on the mend. I am so sorry for what happened to you and your family. I can never repay you for your kindness and what you did for me. I would give you the world if I could and I will forever be indebted to you.

To the doctor who performed my hysterectomy and repaired my prolapses and perineum, I cannot say thank you enough. You gave me the ability to run with my kids again, to laugh and sneeze without peeing all over myself. You made the bleeding finally stop and above all, you listened to me. You believed me and made me feel welcome. You gave me a home that I needed when my world was falling apart. For that, I want to say thank you. I will continue to let the world know that you are an amazing doctor. That you are not one of the doctors that I have mentioned in this memoir. I will continue to sing your praises.

And to the doctor who said he couldn't help me. At first, I was very angry with you. I felt abandoned. I felt like you cast me off onto my own lonely island of mystery diagnoses.

But now, after reflection, I realize you made the right decision. You acknowledged you weren't capable of helping me and communicated that with me. I am thankful that you referred me to someone else, that you weren't too egotistical to keep trying. I want to say thank you for helping me get to my next step in the process.

To the doctor who gave me the courage to go through the surgery because of my golden ticket, I cannot say thank you enough. Your timing saved my life. You may not have ever had the chance to see me but your sense of urgency to review my file and your speed to deliver your opinion was everything to me. You gave me the confidence to know my decision was the right decision and for that I am forever grateful.

To the doctor who actually performed my surgery, you quite literally saved my life. You gave me most of my life back and while I have things that have changed, I am forever grateful. You breathed life back into me. You gave me my smile back, in more ways than one.

You gave me my confidence and will to live back. You believed me and listened to me. You heard me in a way that so many others refused. You acknowledged my concerns and validated me. You trusted that I knew my body and didn't fail me. You will forever be in my heart. I will shout from the rooftops your name. I will make sure that anyone who is like me knows you are available.

Thank you, thank you, thank you.

To the amazing doctor who diagnosed me with Ehlers-Danlos, POTS, and MCAS... THANK YOU.

You provided me with a diagnosis that was imperative for my future health care. While there may be no treatment plan for Ehlers-Danlos, now I have a reason for most of my pain and odd health concerns. You helped put all of the puzzle pieces together so that I could make sense of it all. You treated me with compassion and empathy. You heard me. You

*validated my concerns and sought out ways
to help me. You gave me treatment options for
the things I can control. You sat with me for
over 2 hours, explaining everything to me in
detail. You gave me your time, your heart and
your soul. For that I am forever grateful.
Thank you.*

*To the doctor who validated my collarbone,
thank you. I have gone over a year and a half
with severe collarbone pain and been ignored.
I have been told that there is nothing wrong,
over and over. I have been told that they
could feel something was wrong externally
but on imaging, everything looked "fine",
until you.*

*You looked deeper. You went above and
beyond. You looked for the rare. You treated
me with kindness and respect. You were
compassionate when I cried in front of you
out of sheer exhaustion from not being heard.
You allowed me to wear my heart on my
sleeve without telling me that depression and
anxiety were my issue.*

*If it wasn't for you I would still be in pain
with no reason as to why. I have treatment*

options now. I have a way to correct the pain, besides medication. For that, I am so grateful.

Each and every single one of you gave me my voice back. You helped to turn the light back on. Your compassion, empathy and will to help are what gave me the strength that I needed to not only heal, but to write this. You gave me the power to be able to help others around me and spread positivity around the world.

You gave me a chance to spend time with my wife and kids. Quality time... You gave me the chance to live without being in severe pain 24/7. You reminded me that I was allowed to have both mental health and physical health, without the other influencing my issues.

I hope that each and every one of you keep the flame that is deep inside of your heart. I hope that each and every one of you has a beautiful and wonderful life. I hope that every one of your patients sing your name with praise. You deserve the world and back. I love you all.

TO ALL OTHER DOCTORS IN THIS WORLD:

I know in my heart that there are good doctors in this world. I know from experience that there are doctors who want to make a change and value patient care in the highest regard. I know that there are doctors out there that would cross oceans and lands to ensure that patients were properly treated.

And to those of you that fit that description, I want to say thank you, on behalf of every one of us Zebra's who are living a health nightmare. We owe you our worlds for taking care of us and seeing past the status quo. It is your will to continue searching, that gave us our lives back, even if it was just a fragment.

To the doctors that felt guilt reading this, it is entirely possible to change your path at any time. We as evolving humans have the ability to divert our path onto a new one. It's one of the only perks to humanity at this point.

My intentions are not to come across as a know-it-all or like I have any idea of how to be a doctor, because I certainly do not. I have absolutely no medical background at all.

My intentions are to show you that there is a drastic difference from the patients' perspective of what a good doctor and a bad doctor looks like according to how the doctor treats us.

Our lives are in the palm of your hands. You have full control over OUR health. We have no ability to control our own health or manage it outside of diet, exercise and lifestyle choices (vitamins, etc.)

When you make the decision to ignore our concerns, to refuse to hear what we are saying to us, you ultimately decide our fate in a negative way.

All I ask is that you step outside of your box, that you step outside of what is the "norm" and view us as humans, humans that are crying and screaming for you to help. Humans that are desperate for someone to hear us. Humans that are steadily falling apart before our eyes, living a nightmare that we can't wake up from.

I want you to re-analyze your belief that weight, anxiety and depression are the only *things that can cause issues. I want you to see that there are zebras among the horses and if you refuse to look closely, you will miss them, every single day.*

I do not expect perfection, I expect persistence. I expect a doctor who will not stop until they find the answers that are needed. I expect a doctor who will fight and advocate for us. I expect a doctor who is compassionate, empathetic and kind.

I expect a doctor who continues to educate themselves day in and day out.

We need doctors who aren't afraid to admit that they don't know everything. A doctor who isn't scared to say that they need to do more research or reach out to other practicing professionals around them.

We need doctors who would be willing to stand up with us and fight for their ability to change our healthcare.

I know that doctors face their own battles, face their own obstacles in this world. I am not naive enough to believe that every doctor who refuses to dig deeper does so because they don't want to. I know that insurance companies and laws restrict your ability to look harder, at times.

But I expect that to be a motivation to make a change, the fuel to start a fire that this world needs to see. We need to revolutionize and revamp the entire healthcare industry before it's too late.

If we stand up together, patients and medical professionals alike, then we are stronger. We are unified and determined to see a change. All it takes is one micro piece of rock moving to create and cause an avalanche.

If every single one of us took a stand and refused to be silenced, we could move mountains, together.

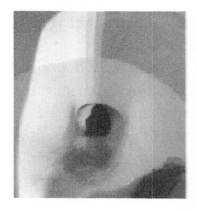

Another massive clot from a day I was at work before I had to stop working.

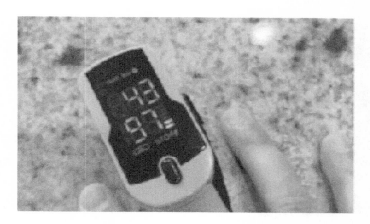

My heart rate right after almost passing out from bending over to grab a laundry basket.

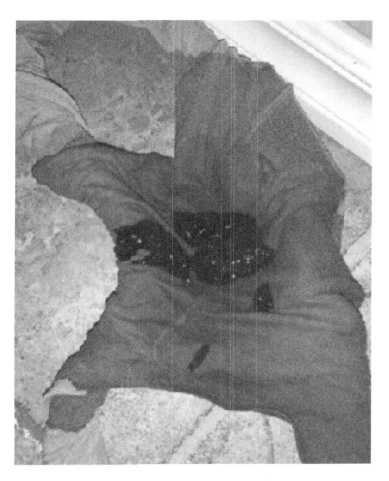

The blood clot from the night I woke up covered in my own blood. The darker portions of my underwear is all blood.

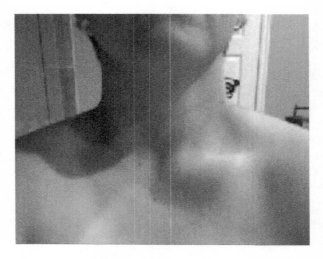

My left collarbone protruding from superior subluxation.

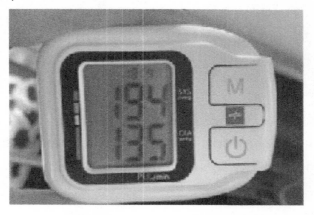

My BP before I went to the hospital for chest pain that felt like someone had my heart in a meat grinder.

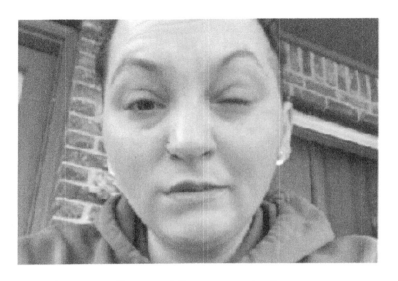

My face swollen and flaring up before surgery.
iPhones flip the photo so this is still my left side.

This patient presents today with the stigmata of a recent fusion of the cervical vertebrae and a release of the pressure of Chiari Syndrome. On examination she has a Beighton score of 9/9 and five of the required secondary findings to support a diagnosis of Ehlers-Danlos syndrome, either Joint Hypermobility, or Vascular type. Her family history is significant enough, with aunts, uncles, father and grandfather having symptoms to suggest a high risk for Vascular EDS.

The disease is based on a fundamental defect in collagen which is the protein glue that holds the body together. It is responsible for the Chiari Malformation and Cranio Cervical Instability, it is responsible for the defect in her clavicle restructuring and also her Postural Orthostatic Tachycardia Syndrome. It is the reason behind her multiple pelvic surgeries and PCOS. She bears the stigmata of Mast Cell Activation Syndrome.

I have discussed this condition in length with her. It is genetic in origin and constitutes a serious medical condition as defined by the Americans with Disabilities Act. I do not expect her to go into remission, but we will help to manage her symptoms and ameliorate her pain and distress in the future.

The letter from my Ehlers Danlos doctor for all of my other physicians. I provided this to my disability company but because Ehlers Danlos is a subjective diagnosis (Unless it's vascular or genetically able to be tested) they refused to acknowledge it as an actual disability. I have removed all identifying information from the letter for both myself and my treating doctor.

And to my kiddos when you are old enough to read this...

It was because you three beautiful souls that I never gave up. It was your little chuckles and contagious laughs that kept a smile on my face. It was watching you grow and change that kept me distracted from the chaos that was becoming life.

I am so incredibly proud of the three of you. I am so proud of the humans you are becoming. The amount of empathy that you all carry deep in your hearts, reminds me that there are good people in this world, kind people.

I know in my heart that the three of you will go far in life. You can and will become whatever you set your mind to. Never let someone steal your sunshine. Never let someone rain on your parade.

Always be the colorful and vibrant humans that you are. Be who you want to be, as long as whoever you want to be isn't against the law, and never give up on your goals and dreams.

You three will leave an imprint on this world. I know in my heart that you will all take steps toward making this planet a better place to be. I love you all with every single piece of my heart.

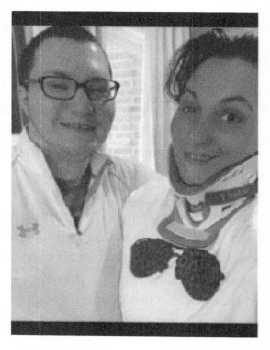

My brother and I while my family was here in Tulsa, helping me recover. I will always be impressed by your ability to light up a room. I love you so much! Your laugh and radiant personality motivate me to always share happiness and positivity. I envy your ability to make someone feel loved and appreciated! I miss your hugs every single day. Never forget how special you are to every single person that meets you!

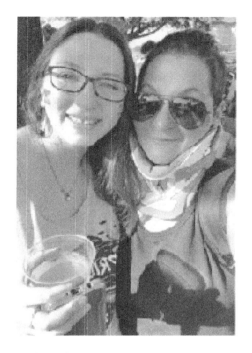

My sister and I at pride (That's just water because it was hotter than Satan's penis outside.)

I was so happy to share this moment with her. She is one of my biggest supporters and I love her for it! You will do absolutely amazing things with your life and I am so incredibly proud of the woman you are becoming! You impress and motivate me every single day without even knowing it. Keep going and never give up. You will soar above the world and fly with your wings extended.

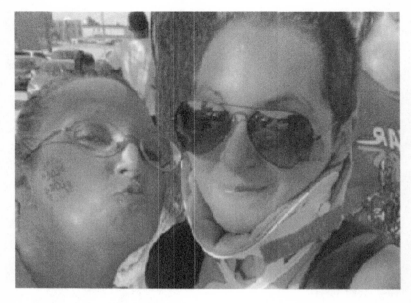

At the Tulsa Pride Festival with family and friends. This is my mom. I was so proud that she came with us. Time can heal wounds and change people. I love you mom! I appreciate the time you took to come to Tulsa and help me through one of the most difficult times of my life. I am thankful for where our relationship is now and how much closer we have grown together!

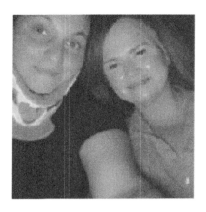

As my vows said, "Rachel, my best friend, my partner in crime, my soulmate, my forever…I love you with all of my heart, with an infinite love deep inside of my soul. You light my soul on fire and keep it blazing. I crave waking up next to you, I crave your touch, your heart. I cherish our memories, our future, the life we have built together. You are my forever and always. You are the missing puzzle piece I have always searched for… You turned my dark days into light. I promise to always love you, to cherish you, to protect you. I promise to always be your shelter in the storms and to be your warmth in the cold. I promise to be your sunrise after the dark and to hold you close. I promise to comfort you and encourage you when you need it. I promise that in both sickness and health I will always be there, I will hold you even if you cannot hold yourself. I will never let a day go by that I don't tell you how absolutely in love with you I am. I promise to always put you and our babies first. I promise to always be the best version of myself I can be for you and for our family. I promise to always keep swimming, to always keep fighting even if things get hard. I promise to love you until we are old and chasing each other with our walkers. I promise to support you through anything and everything and to always work as a team. You are the first thing I want to see when I open my eyes and the absolute last thing I want to feel when I fall asleep. You are my everything and so much more. I cannot simply put into words how lucky I am that in all of the people on this planet, the key to your heart was placed in my possession. I love you Rachel Elise with every single part of my being and I can't wait to spend the rest of my life with you. I cannot wait to create more lasting memories and to build more of our life together one brick at a time. You are my soul mate. My happiness…My one true love.

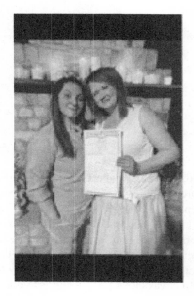

My wedding day, 3-3-22, one of the best days of my life… I got to marry my best friend, my partner in crime, the woman who makes my skies bright and beautiful.

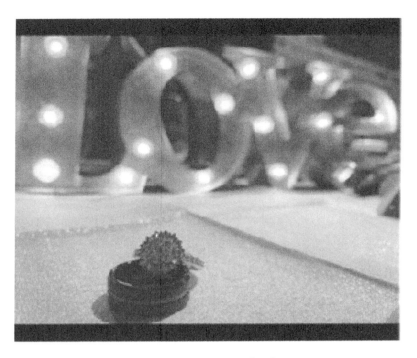

Love can cure any pain that we feel.

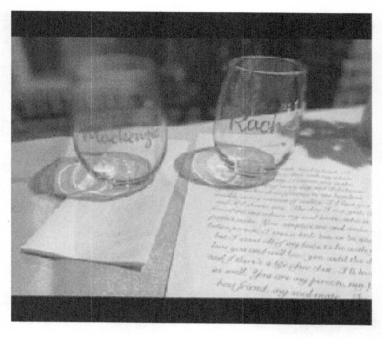

Our vows. Words that poured from our souls onto paper.

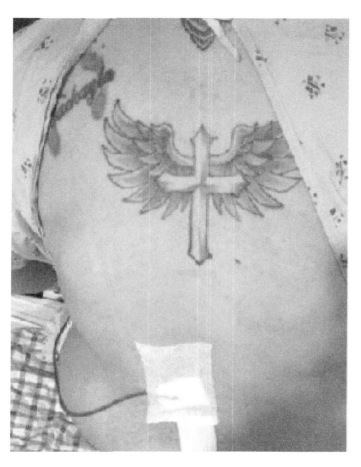

After my L5-S1 PLIF spinal fusion surgery in 2017

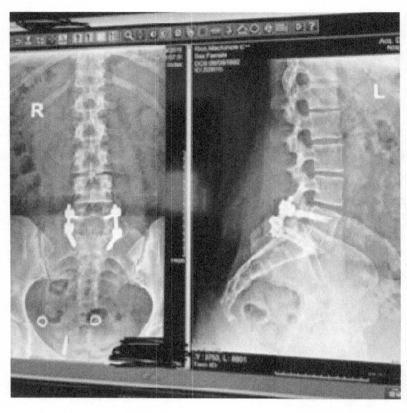

X-Ray post op spinal surgery.

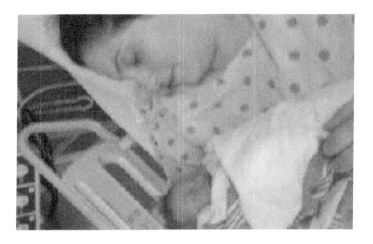

March 25, 2011- The morning I gave birth to my daughter.

And to myself…

Never ever give up. Never ever stop shouting from the rooftops about medical reform and advocacy. No matter how hard things get or how many people tell you to stifle your voice, do not listen. Continue to stand up for those who have not found their strength yet.

Continue to be there for those who are lost and need a hand. Never lose your heart. Never let the world change you, even if it becomes hard.

Just because you have been healed in some ways, just because you have answers, does not mean your journey is over.

It is just the beginning…

I love me.

Never forget that.

MACKENZIE RICE

Self-Published Author of 'Chasing Fear' on Amazon

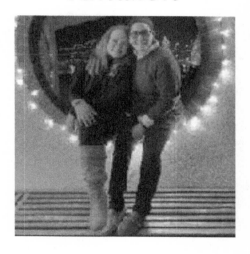

(Bonus points if you can find Rachel's other leg haha.)

"Life can be undeniably the most rewarding and most painful experience we have ever gone through. The lens we choose to view our lives from determines whether we fail or thrive."- Mackenzie

For legal purposes, I have no medical training, nor do I want anyone to believe I do. I am not suggesting anyone raid a doctors' office or commit any violent acts against any medical professional. I am not and will not ever promote violence to any human being, ever.

My sole intentions for this memoir are to help others like myself and to provide hope for the future.

I wish no ill harm on anyone.

*Not everyone's situation will result like mine but if you are experiencing similar symptoms, I do suggest you continue to seek medical care and refuse to back down until you are acknowledged.**

Made in the USA
Las Vegas, NV
21 March 2023

69472895R00135